Love Master

Ricardo Sanchez

DEDICATION

To Anya, a wonderful Daimon
who has enlightened my life

CHAPTERS

INTRODUCTION

Love has always been seen as something possessed by the ego.

Freud , the father of psychoanalysis, disputes this by arguing that since the human psyche is not rational, there is no omnipotent reason that controls the will that determines reasons.

Plato was the first to take an interest in the rules of reason and the abysses of madness. He used the term "madness" to describe an experience of the soul that defies any attempt to fix it and put it in order.

The human psyche is indeed not rational, but something that bumbles along. Love is not something that the ego possesses, but rather something that disposes of the ego, something that divides it and leads it out of the center of its ego.

This is not a book that relies on scripted pick-up lines, seduction tactics or calculated strategies to "find love" with someone.

Our goal is to empower you to master the art of love.

Understanding the psychology behind human relationships is the foundation, but it's your unique charisma and authenticity that will make you shine.

As we delve into the next chapters, each designed to guide you through specific aspects of love and seduction, remember: you are the creator of your own destiny and called to action by your daimon. .

In a philosophical context, the term "'daimon' does not refer to a supernatural being, demon as the English word might suggest. Instead, it is used to describe an inner voice, an inner divine guide or guiding spirit that the Greek philosopher Socrates believed spoke to him.

The daimonion (the term for the inner voice or divine sign) is a kind of spiritual guide that warned him when he was about to make a mistake or a wrong decision, not a source of knowledge per se, not a mystical concept, but rather a source of moral insight, a deep intuition, a compass to embrace one's true nature and uniqueness, which requires the ability to love oneself.

"LOVE MASTER" is a guide to unleashing your potential, to free your daimon.

The path of love begins within.

Chapter by chapter, we guide you through the transformation into the best version of yourself.

It's not about conforming to societal expectations or adopting a false persona.

No, it's about embracing your authenticity, amplifying your strengths and addressing your weaknesses with an awareness of your own imperfections as part of a [non]perfect universe, a journey to face your own darkness and inner demons and then ultimately find the light of love.

LOVE MASTER

1 DESIRE

In the mainstream or notorious "pop" imagination, "love"
is an illusion of emotional stability, a romantic fiction of
honey and sugar that movies serve up to the masses, so we
tend to fall in love due to cultural
(mis)education, we tend to identify the search for love with
this kind of drama as a goal.
It's actually the opposite.
This concept that erases the longing when we reach the
goal, we should call it "romance" is not really love, because
true love is indeed the pinnacle of desire.

Desire demands novelty, mystery and danger, it should be
able to combat time, routine and familiarity.
In fact, looking for security and stability leads love to its
downfall because it fails to embrace the adventure,
excitement and sense of risk that fuel its passion.
Desire does not actually know what it wants;

It's an unfounded act that everyone finds in unbearable
gestures, like an uncontrolled force breaking into stability
and order, as we can see our "daimon" in action.

Unknown forces guide the daimon on the path to full personal fulfillment, just as desire has irrational origins, according to the intrinsic nature of the being that does not follow logic and guides our actions driven by unstoppable passion; just think of the crazy gestures performed in the frenzy of desire for a loved one.

Unlike "romantic love", which seeks to build stability, desire is a movement towards a point of loss.
Contrary to all logic, desire plays, but its game has no rules, because rules are the negation of the game itself.
In the game of desire, actions do not respond to a calculation or a cause-effect logic in a "trade" conception, in fact desire only knows theft and the gift.
For this reason, love, which strives for stability, tends to extinguish desire.

Hence the success of online love… where the fantasy of unleashing one's desire with a person who is not there or unavailable offers not only the opportunity to explore the forbidden and precarious, but also the opportunity to fantasize about the forbidden.
But not everyone is ready to fully embrace the lure of the unknown.

Understanding the EGO

We all use the first person pronoun: "I", which eliminates the need to mention our specific names. Instead of saying "I, Ricardo, am going out"," it's easier to express it as "I am going out" Although my name is Ricardo, it's more comfortable to say "I" because it makes everything seem simple and clear.
But when it comes to the name, it serves as a substitute for the identity— that defines who I am.

This is where things get a little complicated. The question arises: Do I really know who I am? The typical answer might be that I know — I am an engineer, a sports fan, a teacher, a husband. This answer may seem convincing, but it falls short. How can I formulate it? Quite simply: even if I change jobs or change my social role, I continue to use the pronoun "I"

Defining your own identity is a major challenge.

We usually confuse identity with identification, but these are different concepts. I can identify with my body, my job, my family status, my hobbies, my beliefs, my ideas and my feelings, but none of these aspects define who I am. They are subject to change, while the core of my being remains constant.

In reality, I am a center of consciousness and will characterized by the uniqueness of my daimon, which observes my body, thoughts and emotions as I observe them.

Building on this concept, which is inspired by Asian psychology, we find a powerful technique known as the disidentification exercise.

The repetition of the formula proposed by this exercise reveals the truth of its basis. For example, the realisation: "I am really not my anger, for I can observe it, just as I can observe the clouds in the sky." When we engage in this linguistic exercise, we discover that the emotions that once dominated us gradually lose their hold on our inner self.

Everything we identify with dominates us.

What does "dominate us" mean?

It means that our whereabouts are no longer under our sole control. When we claim: "I have decided to go to the movies"," we are perpetuating an untruth. The actual truth is far from it: "An emotion, the origin of which eludes me, emerged in me and forced me to believe that I had made the decision to go to the movies. It was not me, but an emotion of unknown origin that decided on my behalf."

Coming to terms with this reality is harrowing. It forces us to fundamentally change our previous self-perception, which can be extremely painful. This is the reason for the resistance that many show to such concepts.
However, if we want to walk the path of love, a journey that requires an ever more precise understanding of our inner processes, we must go beyond this point.

"**Gnòthi seautòn",**" proclaimed the oracle of Delphi.

Know yourself, and in doing so you will recognize both yourself and the divine within you. Someone who lacks self-knowledge behaves like a puppet — mechanically, manipulated by the strings held by others. Another way to emphasise the linguistic deception of the pronoun "I" is to assume that it refers to a single individual. Otherwise, one would use the pronoun "we". In reality, as we all experience, there are moments of inner conflict. One part of us desires one thing, while another part longs for something different or even opposite. Basically, our personality is divided into different components, different sub-personalities, different selves, each with its own will. The perception of an inner conflict is an everyday phenomenon. But the prevailing notion suggests that it is temporary, an exceptional disturbance that occurs and resolves itself. In reality, conflict is the norm, not the exception. The plurality of egos and subpersonalities is a fundamental aspect of human existence. As Eugen Bleuler, Jung's mentor, noted more than a century ago, we are born with some degree of schizophrenia, and if we are lucky, one part gradually gains dominance to dominate the personality and control the remaining smaller parts. Bleuler illuminates the concept of self-governance, an essential idea for navigating the often opaque realms of the psyche. To illustrate this, the human model includes three levels of the unconscious: the lower, middle and upper unconscious. The lower unconscious harbours subpersonalities and their conflicts, similar to the pathogenic unconscious in psychoanalysis. The middle unconscious, which is easily accessible, houses the dominant ego with which we normally identify. Finally, the upper unconscious, which is neglected by classical psychoanalysis, is the abode of the true self or soul — a reservoir of wisdom, developed principles, values and resources.

Self-realisation is about tapping into this potential, divinizing one's human existence and merging with the divine, humanity, all living beings and existence as a whole. This profound task requires raising one's own state of consciousness from the lower levels, which are characterised by an intense identification with the subpersonalities originating from childhood, to the highest levels, where absolute freedom and creativity prevail. This state corresponds to the consciousness of "Jesus Christ" for Christians and "Samadhi" for Eastern philosophies. Only at this level, which is only reached by a few saints or illuminati, can one overcome the mechanisms of the lower psyche, such as mood swings and mental stagnation. This means that the vast majority of humanity struggles all their lives with their ego, a force that often stands in the way of personal and collective well-being.

Desire is Infatuation

The distinction between love and infatuation can be compared to the concept of the ego, showing how each emotional experience is related to different aspects of self-perception and interpersonal dynamics:

Reality vs. Idealization

Love: love is based on a realistic understanding of the other person including strengths and weaknesses. This means accepting the person as they are, acknowledging imperfections and building a connection based on shared experiences.

Infatuation (ego): Infatuation, which corresponds to the ego's desire for an idealized self-perception, can lead to an idealized image being projected onto the other person. The person in love may see the object of their affection through a filtered lens, emphasizing the positive qualities and overlooking the weaknesses, similar to how the ego attempts to maintain an idealized self-image.

Connection vs. Impressions

Love: love involves a deep emotional connection characterized by understanding, empathy and commitment. It goes beyond superficial impressions and allows individuals to connect on a deep level that goes beyond initial attraction.

Infatuation (ego): Infatuation, which corresponds to the ego's preoccupation with superficial appearances, can be triggered by immediate physical attraction or external qualities. The person in love may focus on certain qualities or appearances without looking at the deeper aspects of the other person's character.

Emotional maturity vs. Emotional satisfaction

Love: Love is associated with emotional maturity, where individuals overcome challenges, communicate effectively and develop each other. It requires a willingness to invest in a long-term, committed relationship.

Infatuation (ego): Infatuation reflects the ego's desire for immediate emotional gratification and may focus more on the intense feelings and excitement associated with initial attraction. The person in love may prioritize the thrill of infatuation over the long-term emotional maturity required for a committed relationship.

Response to challenges vs. fragility in adversity

Love: love tends to weather challenges, with couples working together to overcome difficulties. The commitment and shared history in love provide a foundation to overcome adversity.

Infatuation (ego): Infatuation reflects the fragility of the ego when faced with challenges, and can be difficult to withstand difficulties. When the initial thrill wears off, the infatuated feelings can fade, much like the ego can falter when faced with setbacks in its idealized self-image.

Mutual growth vs. Self-realization

Love: Love includes mutual growth, where both individuals contribute to each other's personal development; in the most genuine egoistic meaning, love for oneself admits the ability to improve the other. It goes beyond self-actualization and emphasizes the growth and well-being of the relationship as a whole.

Infatuation (ego): Infatuation, which is similar to the ego's pursuit of self-realization, may focus more on personal gratification and the immediate emotional high associated with infatuation. The person in love may prioritize their own emotional experience over the broader growth of the relationship.

Infatuation VS Love

Desire (infatuation): Imagine a scenario in which someone is infatuated with another person's physical appearance or charisma. The attraction is intense and is primarily driven by a desire for closeness, passion or novelty.

Love (committed love): In contrast, consider a couple that has been together for many years. Their love has developed beyond purely physical attraction. It involves shared experiences, mutual understanding and a commitment to each other's well-being that goes beyond the initial spark of desire.

Desire (material possession): Imagine someone who longs for a luxury car. The desire is based on the allure of owning something prestigious that offers status or pleasure.

Love (Emotional Attachment): Now think of a parent's love for their child. This love is not based on material possessions, but on a deep emotional connection, a bond that goes beyond material desires and is supported by care, nurturing and an innate sense of responsibility.

Desire (short-term attraction): Imagine a situation in which two people are attracted to each other at a party. Their interaction is driven by a temporary attraction, perhaps triggered by appearance or shared interests at that moment.

Love (Long-term commitment): Compare this to a couple celebrating their 50th wedding anniversary. Their love has survived challenges and developed into a deep connection that goes beyond fleeting attraction. It is a testament to long-term commitment, understanding and shared life experiences.

Desire (self-congratulation): Imagine someone seeking a chance encounter for personal pleasure. desire is focused on satisfying immediate physical or emotional needs without making a long-term commitment.

Love (Selfless Caring): In contrast, imagine a caregiver supporting a sick partner. Love in this scenario involves selfless acts that put the other person's well-being above one's own desires. It goes beyond personal gratification and leads to a deeper level of commitment and care.

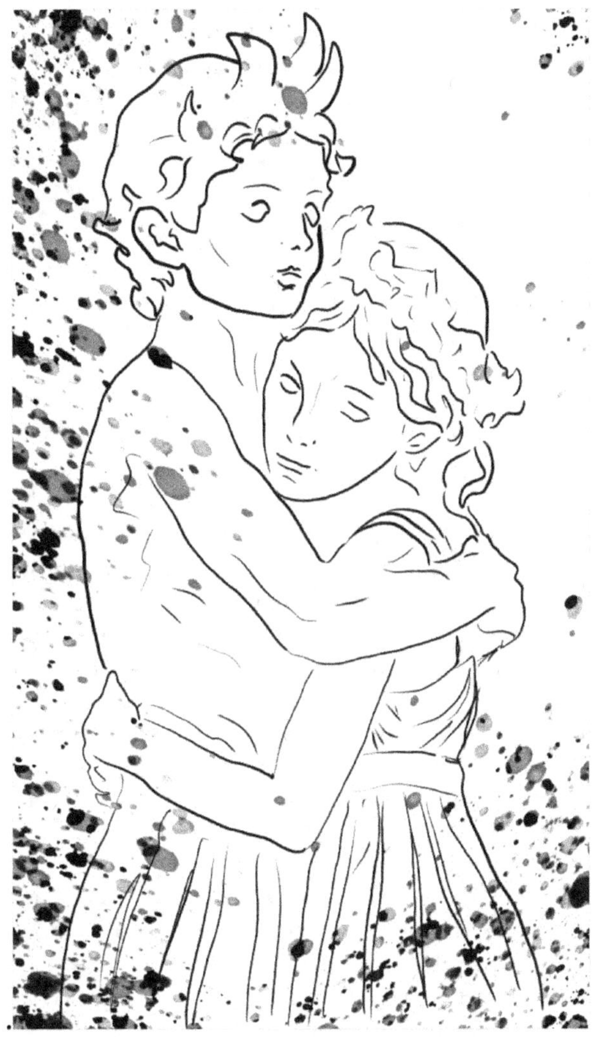

Desire

While desire involves attraction and wanting, love extends beyond the initial spark to encompass deep emotional connections, commitment, selfless care.

2 UNCONSCIOUS

The unconscious mind can be likened to an unexplored territory that holds the key to understanding our deepest desires and fears. Freud's pioneering exploration of the realm beneath the surface of our thoughts and emotions unveiled a complex language that influences our actions, often without our conscious awareness. Understanding the unconscious is an endeavor that requires deciphering the intricate language of our hidden motivations. Our unconscious minds house desires that are often buried and obscured from our conscious minds. These desires can shape our perceptions, decisions, and interactions like dormant seeds. Learning to master the unconscious mind can help us unearth these hidden longings and transform them into a powerful tool for personal growth. Being aware of our own desires, as well as the desires of others, can help us navigate the intricacies of human connection with ease.

To master the unconscious is to gain a profound understanding of the mechanisms that drive human behavior. Armed with this knowledge, you become an irresistible force—a maestro driving emotions and influencing the thoughts and desires of those around you. The ability to decode the unspoken language of the unconscious provides a strategic advantage in the pursuit of personal and interpersonal goals.

As you become attuned to the whispers of your own hidden desires, you gain a clarity that extends beyond the surface of conscious thought. This self-awareness becomes a beacon, illuminating the path to personal growth and empowerment.

Understanding the unconscious is not merely a solitary endeavor on a personal level.

By recognizing the unconscious desires of others, you forge bonds that transcend the superficial, creating connections based on an authentic understanding of shared motivations. The mastery of the unconscious allows you to navigate the subtle nuances of social dynamics, establishing yourself as a captivating and influential presence.

Alienation with the other for self-love ends either in assimilation with the loved one, which leads to the loss of one's identity, or in possession of the loved one, with the tendency to exclude it from the world.

Lovers call this mutual love identification, and this renunciation of oneself and one's freedom does not only express a relationship of dependence but a real condition of alienation.

Maintenance in love of one's autonomy not only avoids identification with the loved one but also allows for self-recovery.

Personal interests:

Understanding one's unconscious desires and motivations allows an individual to navigate the complex landscape of attraction. By recognizing what truly attracts them to others, they can align their actions with genuine intentions, fostering authentic connections.

Managing Insecurities:

Self-awareness helps individuals identify and manage insecurities that may hinder their ability to connect with others. By acknowledging and addressing these insecurities, individuals can approach seduction with confidence, authenticity, and a reduced fear of rejection.

Recognizing Patterns of Attraction:

Unconscious patterns often shape attraction. By becoming aware of recurring patterns in the types of individuals one is drawn to, an individual can make informed choices about potential partners and understand the deeper reasons behind their attractions.

Adjusting Communication Styles:

Understanding one's unconscious communication style is essential in seduction. It involves recognizing non-verbal cues, body language, and the impact of past experiences on current interactions. Adjusting communication styles based on this awareness enhances the effectiveness of conveying interest and establishing a connection.

Addressing Unresolved Issues:

Unresolved issues from the past can significantly impact present interactions. Self-awareness allows individuals to identify and address these issues, preventing them from negatively influencing the seduction process. Emotional healing contributes to healthier and more fulfilling connections.

Cultivating Emotional Intelligence:

Seduction involves a nuanced understanding of emotions, both one's own and those of others. Developing emotional intelligence through self-awareness enables individuals to navigate the emotional complexities of attraction, fostering deeper connections based on empathy and understanding.

Very often people do not show themselves to the world as they really are, a phenomenon that Carl Jung describes in his shadow psychology, but even more surprising is that many of them are not even what they believe they are; this happens because most people fear expressing their true nature, especially those parts that might be seen as unacceptable by society. To avoid the discomfort that this entails, many people divide themselves into a conscious and an unconscious part: in the conscious part, they create an ideal image of themselves based on those aspects of their past that they consider acceptable, and in the unconscious part, they repress those aspects that they consider negative. According to Jung, this repressed part of the personality is known as the shadow; without shadow integration, a person cannot realize their full potential.

She is therefore left with an incomplete and fragmented version of herself, condemned to a life of regret rather than a fully realized life.

To better illustrate the concept, let's take the example of a musician who, after having composed some melodies, is convinced that he is an exceptional musician...

One day, his friends invite him to join a musical group that meets regularly to play and compose music together. This makes him anxious; by joining the group, he risks discovering that he is not the extraordinary musician he thought he was. Faced with this situation, he can choose two paths: the first is to avoid confrontation with his shadow by refusing to join the group; in doing so, he maintains the illusion of being a great musician but loses the opportunity to truly grow and improve. The second option is to face his shadow by joining the group. This may reveal that he is not as talented as he thought, but it also offers him the chance to discover new aspects and potential of his musical talent.

Therefore, confronting one's shadow can be painful in the short term, but it is a fundamental step for authentic personal growth. In the real world, we can improve and make our dreams come true, while a life lived in an illusion only leads to a tragic end. The key to a satisfying life begins with the acceptance and integration of our shadow, welcoming even the less pleasant aspects of ourselves.

This allows us to reach our maximum potential; if, however, we reject our shadow by choosing only the aspects of our personality that we like and repress those that we fear, we remain incomplete and dissatisfied, living a life of regrets. The choice therefore is to accept reality with all its ups and downs or take refuge in an illusion that, although comforting, prevents us from living fully.

In Jungian terms, will you accept your shadow or continue to reject it?

Narcissism and Toxic love

Narcissism stems from the experience of being humiliated—feeling powerless in the face of others' dominance without the strength to rebel. In response, the narcissist decides to accumulate as much power as possible, aiming to avoid future humiliation. This decision is attributed to the "mask," the constructed personality that governs our sense of self. Once in power, this persona doesn't hesitate to endorse the ego's tendencies toward retaliation, vindictiveness, and arrogance, staying within the acceptable bounds set by the social context.

For the narcissist, the mask serves the crucial function of regulating the excesses of the lower self. The lower self, driven by a sense of omnipotence and grandiosity, lacks self-imposed limits and could lead the individual to self-destructive behavior impacting others. However, the mask acts as a restraint—a control mechanism—distinct from forcing a complete shift in direction.

It's worth noting that our culture, at its core, is deeply infused with narcissistic assumptions and foundations. In essence, we exist in an environment that promotes this distorted perspective. Leonardo Boff articulates this sentiment, highlighting that the prevailing ethics in today's society are utilitarian and anthropocentric. The prevalent belief is that everything revolves around the human being, positioning them as the lord and master of nature—seeing nature as existing solely to fulfill human needs and desires. This underlying worldview tends to foster violence and the domination of both others and the natural world.

From the viewpoint of some authors, like Alexander Lowen, narcissism is believed to have roots deeper than just the inhibition of exhibitionism. It is suggested that, at its core, narcissism emerges from a profound experience during childhood where the child undergoes the distressing humiliation of being overpowered by someone deriving sadistic pleasure from subjugating them. In this scenario, the child is left with no option but to endure the suffering, lacking the strength to respond. However, the imprint of this humiliation is etched vividly in the child's psyche, an indelible mark that remains unforgettable.

Consequently, a desire for retribution takes root—a drive to dominate others and subject them to humiliation. This aligns with a general principle that posits a tendency to reciprocate what one has experienced. The need for revenge becomes a way to regain a sense of power and control, driven by the lingering memory of the initial humiliation endured during childhood.

Indeed, within the narcissist, there resides a sense of shame—the feeling of being caught engaging in something deemed inappropriate. What prompts this shame? It stems from the inherent desire to perform and be admired, a need that is entirely natural in young children. However, as this need is suppressed, it finds its way into the unconscious, where it remains stagnant and undeveloped. Consequently, this unmet need persists into adulthood, at times manifesting intensely and dramatically.

The inability to receive the acknowledgment and approval sought becomes a source of renewed narcissistic anger, fueling the lower self. To shield against potential humiliation, the mask the narcissist wears opts for a path of power and arrogance. This choice, while protecting against shame, inadvertently obstructs a significant portion of the narcissist's emotional experiences. They become incapable of feeling and expressing sadness and fear, perceiving these emotions as indicators of weakness. In alignment with the mask, the emotion that can be felt and openly displayed is anger, viewed as an expression of power.

Another element contributing to narcissism involves the direct influence of one of the parents, inducing the child to believe they are special. Instead of being accepted for their true identity, the child is encouraged to identify with a grandiose image—not for who they are, but for what they can represent or pretend to be. Initially, this satisfies the child's exhibitionistic needs, and they easily fall into this enticing trap. However, the child soon realizes that the parent wielding this influence has significant power over them. This parent can either confirm or disconfirm the grandiose image with which the child has identified, holding control over it at their discretion. The child feels entirely at the mercy of this parent, and thus, the dynamic of submission and arrogance, foundational to narcissism, is established.

Moreover, as the child identifies with the grandiose image, a continuous need for confirmation arises to uphold this self-image. However, the child soon discovers that the external world may not consistently provide the narcissistic affirmations they crave. While it might be easy for a child to deceive themselves into thinking they are exceptional, this illusion clashes with reality as they grow older and face reactions from others. What the child fears most is judgment that diminishes them, placing them on the same level as others and toppling them from the pedestal. This fear arises because such judgment threatens to immerse them in depressive feelings of insignificance, weakness, and impotence. To avoid this, the child reacts with anger, seeking to humiliate others, erase them, and thereby strip them of any power over the narcissist. If the other person is nullified or eliminated, they can no longer inflict harm, humiliation, or wounds upon the narcissist. This often explains why narcissists exhibit domineering and sadistic behaviors, with narcissism standing as the root cause of some of the most destructive and ruthless actions that humans may engage in, ranging from torture to genocide.

Individuals with narcissistic tendencies often exhibit pride, arrogance, and vanity. Their response to negative feedback typically involves feelings of anger or shame. It's common for them to frequently criticize the perceived shortcomings of others. Many people describe their interactions with narcissists as marked by a love-hate cycle, where they are drawn in by their charm yet simultaneously exploited.

A pivotal moment in therapy occurs when narcissists allow themselves to tap into feelings of sadness and embrace vulnerability. This shift is crucial as it enables them to recognize that vulnerability doesn't render them weak or susceptible to humiliation. Instead, it becomes a gateway to the richness and warmth of more authentic communication. Fundamentally, they must grasp that true strength doesn't reside in denying emotions and projecting superiority. On the contrary, authentic strength is found in the courage to reveal vulnerability.

Heinz Kohut proposes that the same forces, potentially negative and devoid of humanity, can be channeled for good and evolution once their inherent transformation occurs. The dynamic of the grandiose self and exhibitionism, when successfully resolved, serves as the foundation for robust self-esteem. Individuals learn to believe in themselves and their potential for fulfillment through dedicated efforts in study, work, and commitment. Conversely, unresolved narcissism, marked by excessive pride, poses a significant impediment to this positive trajectory.

In alignment with Asian psychologies, attachment to the self is recognized as a common obstacle on the path of personal evolution. This attachment implies viewing oneself as unique and special, unwilling to relinquish this identity even for the sake of greater happiness. The struggle to abandon oneself, fully trust, and attune to the inner self often finds its roots in this attachment—the belief that one is different and special.

The transformative journey leads individuals to feel an integral part of something more extensive: humanity, all living beings, and the universe. Kohut terms this cosmic narcissism. While Freud considered it a neurotic aspect, Kohut perceives it as an ultimate goal, achievable by very few. In this state, the profound fear of death diminishes as death itself takes on a new meaning—no longer the end and nothingness, but a transformation into something greater.

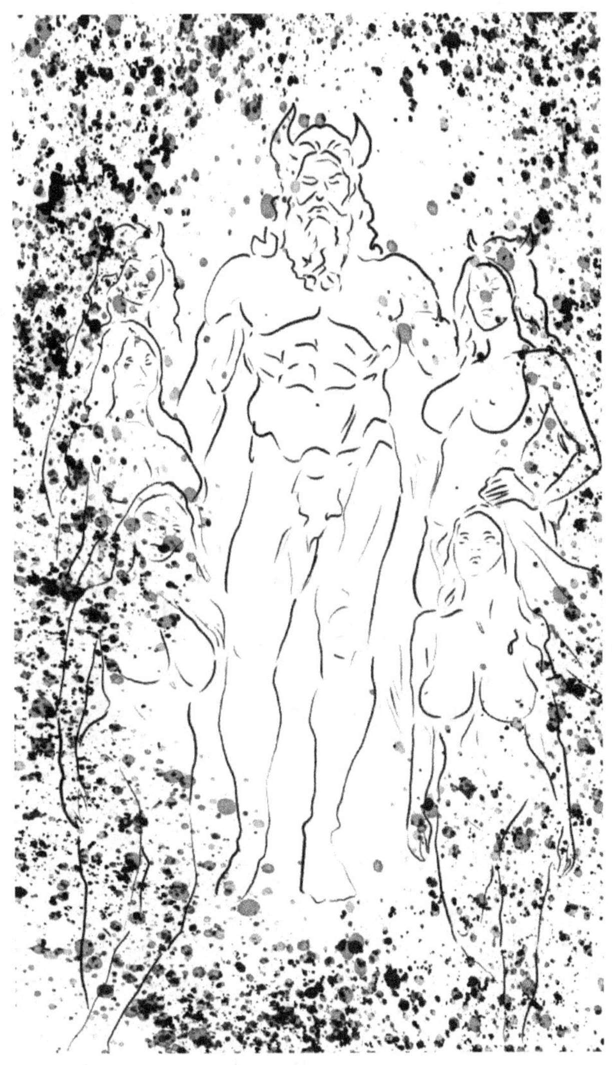

Unconscious

Recognize the inner motivation of your soul in order
to get genuine relationships; embrace your own
shadow brings to full expression and realization.

3 EROS

In Greek mythology, Eros, the god of love and desire, is often described as the son of Poenia (or sometimes Aphrodite) and Poros. Poenia represents the personification of longing or desire, while Poros symbolizes plenty or wealth. Eros, born from this union, embodies the concept of desire and abundance, the intertwining of love and lack, symbolizing the idea that love arises from a state of need. As the mischievous god responsible for igniting passion and love, Eros is typically depicted with a bow and arrows, capable of enchanting both gods and mortals alike. The myth of Eros, born from the union of Poenia and Poros, encapsulates the idea that desire and abundance are intricately connected, influencing the human experience.

In the ancient Greek myth of Eros and Psyche, Psyche's exceptional beauty incites the jealousy of Aphrodite. However, when Eros is tasked with making Psyche fall in love with a wretched creature, he himself falls for her.

Their clandestine love faces trials orchestrated by Aphrodite. Despite Psyche's moment of betrayal and a perilous journey to the underworld, their love triumphs. The gods, moved by their sincerity, grant Psyche immortality, and she and Eros are united in a divine marriage. This enduring myth encapsulates the transformative power of love, from trials to triumphant union.

Each tale, whether it be the tragic romance of Orpheus and Eurydice or the daring exploits of Perseus and Andromeda, is a valuable lesson for the modern seeker of love.

As we explore these myths, let's draw parallels to our own experiences. Consider the challenges faced by Eros and Psyche as metaphors for the obstacles that often arise in modern relationships.

Psyche, the maiden with her mortal vulnerabilities, represents our own human fragilities and imperfections. Eros, the mischievous god of love, embodies the transformative power of passion and connection. Their union, though tested by trials, ultimately reveals the enduring strength of love's invisible threads.

Sigmund Freud, the father of psychoanalysis, introduced the concepts of Eros and Thanatos as fundamental drives shaping human behavior.

Eros is a life drive, a desire for union, construction, and relationships, often represented by sexual drives.

Thanatos is a death drive and therefore a desire for self-destruction or destruction, often represented by man's intrinsic aggressiveness towards his peers.

Freud theorized that the interplay between Eros and Thanatos creates a dynamic tension within the human psyche, influencing thoughts, emotions, and behaviors.

Freud believed that this perpetual struggle between life and death instincts shapes human motivations and behaviors, contributing to the complexities of the human psyche. The Eros-Thanatos duality is integral to Freud's broader psychoanalytic theory, providing insights into the conflicting forces that drive human actions and relationships and the perpetual quest for balance between the constructive and destructive aspects of our existence.

"Eros" by Plato is a concept explored in several of his philosophical dialogues, most notably in the "Symposium." In this dialogue, a group of intellectuals gathers to discuss the nature of love and, specifically, the concept of Eros. Eros, in this context, represents a type of love associated with desire, often romantic or sexual in nature.

Eros Origins

Plato's "Symposium" presents various speeches by different characters, each offering their own perspective on love. Aristophanes, for example, presents a mythological account suggesting that humans were once dual beings powerful androgynous creatures feared by gods, wich were splitted to limit their powers; in so Eros represents a longing for reunion with their lost halves.

According to Aristophanes, Eros arises from a sense of incompleteness and a yearning for unity. The idea is that humans were once whole but were split into two, and Eros is the force that drives them to seek their lost halves, whether in the form of a romantic partner or a deeper connection with another person.

The character Socrates engages in a dialogue with Diotima, a wise woman, who imparts her wisdom on the nature of Eros. Diotima describes Eros not merely as a love for the physical or the beautiful but as a striving for the eternal and the divine. Eros, in this sense, becomes a path toward a higher form of love and knowledge.

Diotima introduces the concept of the "Ladder of Love," which represents a progression from the physical attraction of bodies to the appreciation of beautiful souls and ideas. Ultimately, Eros becomes a means of transcending the material world and attaining a connection with eternal truths.

Plato's Eros is not solely focused on physical attraction but is seen as an educational force. Through love, individuals can be guided toward intellectual and moral improvement.

The lovers, driven by Eros, seeks the betterment of both themselves and their beloved.

Eros, according to Plato, is a force that propels individuals toward the pursuit of beauty and truth. It is not confined to romantic or sexual love but extends to the love of wisdom (philosophy) and the appreciation of eternal and unchanging beauty.

Plato's exploration of Eros in the "Symposium" provides a rich and multifaceted understanding of love, encompassing both the physical and the metaphysical terms.

Eros in modernity

If we are not afraid of words, we can say that madness inhabits Eros, the senses.

Sensuality feels that totality is elusive, that non-sense contaminates sense, and that the possible exceeds the real, opening up a dizzying availability to all the senses.

Of course loss of the senses, with all the fantasies that contribute to it. In sensuality, the game is higher because the goal is not the enjoyment of the ego, but it gets lost in those regions where the words is entrusted to the otherness that we have removed.

Sensuality involves birth and death.

Death of the ego and rebirth in new configurations.

What we call enjoyment of the ego is actually its unraveling because it is permitted the opening to that part of us that we are no longer.

Either you pass through, or the game remains without thickness.

Love does not deny sex (Eros) but makes them revolve around you so that each of us feels like part of your destiny, your "daimon.".

No one actually loves the other, but everyone loves what they have created with it, regardless of the other.

We are irreducibly limited in our daimon realization as a limited particle of an infinite universe.

Eros is violence

Body wildness and love are violent, not good manners:

If a child sees his parents in a love scene, he says that his father and mother are fighting!

In love, there is an essential and genuine dose of aggression due to the suppression of language as a channel of communication, precisely because we are unable to communicate with linguistic mediation, and therefore, at a distance, we have to do a body-to-body which is the violent gesture.

Love is not made of caresses.

Eros involves erotic violence.

Humanity cannot ignore it.

Since we cannot be saved from eroticism because the regime is that of madness, we have established reason, civility, and good manners, from which the whole world of classification takes over. Then we identify "falling in love," "marriage, "and "friendship," which, however, are all surrogate forms of eroticism and can be attributed to a basic human instinct of voluptuousness and murder.

This is love.

In love, we tend to suppress the other; in a paradoxical sense, the sentimental regime is ambivalent, as is madness, the absence of balance, and the meeting of opposites; otherwise, we would talk about reason.

With reason, we can distinguish love from hate according to certain criteria that we set at the level of human behavior to identify what is acceptable or not in a society.But your feelings don't mark that difference. Every person for whom you feel love is also the object of violent hatred.

If you have the ability to deeply explore your feelings for a person, you will discover that what has just been said is true.

We all have a charge of aggression and violence, which we relegate to our unconscious state of ego and which we express in a veiled way in our communication with others, which translates into irony, comments, and complaints, up to that exploit, which is verbal violence observable during a heated confrontation rather than an argument with the partner.

Violence in the erotic context therefore reaches its maximum level.

Love is also hate.

There is no mediation, and there is no good education in love.

Sadism is a parody of the wickedness that exists in love and of its genuine violent component, in light of the fact that all feelings are ambivalent.

The father or mother you love is the same father or mother you hate, the child you love, is the same one you hate.

Love is never univocal and linear; actually it brings with it its negation, just as God is day and night, as Heraclitus states.

Starting from these principles, we have built classifications such as marriage.

If a marriage is based on the principle of erotica, for example, it's gonna fall very soon.

While erotica knows no rules like madness, marriage is based on that principle of long-term commitment and that emotional component aimed at taking care of the other, a rule that ignores the erotic side to embrace a meaning of "love." Deeper, it is made up of rules, like an artistic discipline. We could say that marriage is indeed an art.

Impulse of destruction and self-destruction

Marie-Louise Von Franz , Jung's student, asserts that if the origin of the sexual drive lies in a straightforward pursuit of pleasure, it becomes challenging to repress it effortlessly. However, considering sexuality as a principle of fusion, where one forfeits the sense of self in the other, eradicating individuality, it becomes a force that the delicate barrier of the unconscious safeguarding the ego cannot easily withstand.

From this perspective of awareness, it becomes clear that a genuine impulse toward self-destruction or the dissolution of the ego, revealing one's true self, is, in fact, the authentic and self-centered motivation underlying every sexual relationship. The objective is not a social connection with others but the pursuit of self-discovery.

In essence, authentic sexuality involves the destruction of the ego.

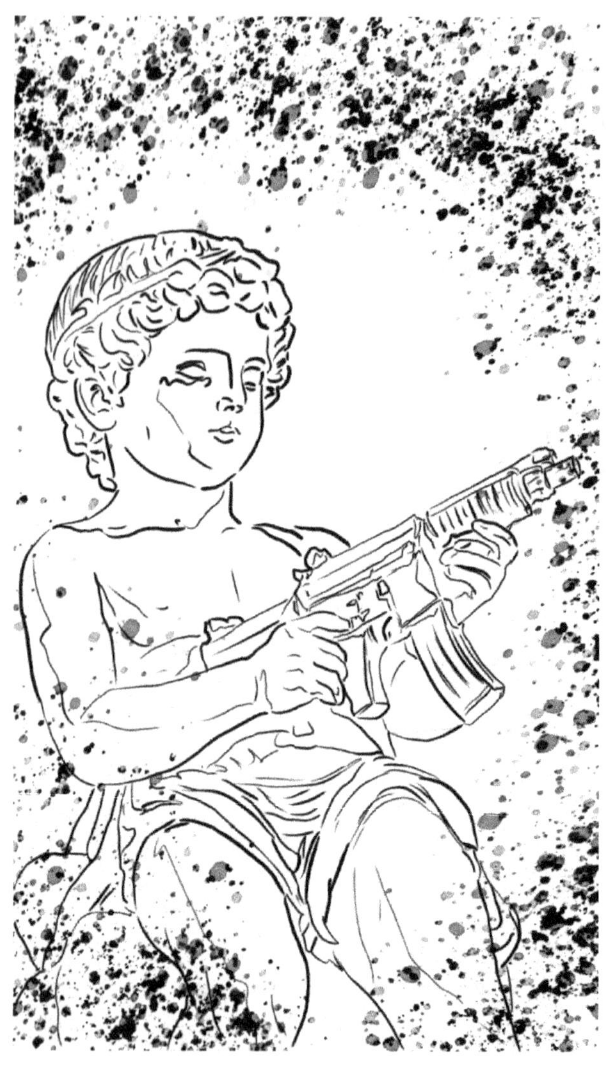

Eros

Love is facing challenges and obstacles, a balance
between passion and restraint, abundance and
scarcity, the essence of human pursuit of fulfillment.

4 SELF LOVE

Break free from societal norms. Freedom in love encourages you to embrace individuality. Celebrate your uniqueness, and let others do the same.

Loving oneself is a prerequisite for loving others. Cultivate self-respect and confidence. A person who loves themselves becomes magnetic to others.

Embracing Imperfection

In the domain of love, flaws are not viewed as shortcomings but rather as unique qualities that enhance the beauty of our connections. As we delve into the practice of accepting imperfections and fostering growth, imagine a garden where each flaw serves as evidence of the genuine love blossoming within.

Freud's theories explored the essence of imperfection within the human mind. Our vulnerabilities, quirks, and distinct traits are the elements that shape our beings. Similar to the introspective journey we undertake, this exploration is a personal voyage, a private dialogue concerning the recognition and appreciation of the imperfections that define our humanity.

Reflect on the virtues of patience and persistence, essential components in nurturing love. Like a gardener tending to delicate flowers, we examine how giving love the necessary time and space enables it to thrive. Drawing from Freud's insights, we understand that love is not an immediate occurrence but a gradual process that, with patience, evolves into a comforting, enduring flame.

Consider imperfection not as a hindrance but as a catalyst for personal and mutual advancement.

Love is not about possession but about the shared journey of growth.

Embrace your imperfections, and your progress journey.

The art of waiting

In the intricate journey of love, patience emerges as a guiding force, steering the course of relationships with deliberate intent. It is an active practice, creating space for understanding and allowing connections to unfold organically. Patience, a virtue often undervalued, acts as the nurturing ground for deeper comprehension, fostering bonds that withstand the tests of time. In quiet moments, where words pause, patience reveals its eloquence, giving emotions the time they need to settle and grow. A dynamic virtue, patience is not passive but a constant motion—a commitment to the journey of love, weathering challenges, and allowing relationships to evolve naturally. In the art of waiting, there is an eloquence in the moments of silence. It is a pause that allows emotions to settle, understanding to blossom, and love to find its voice. The unspoken dialogue becomes as meaningful as words, and the quietude becomes a canvas where emotions are painted with the brushstrokes of time.

Patience becomes the catalyst for enduring connections, and the reward is found in the profound understanding that comes from waiting gracefully, building connections that endure with depth, resilience, and the timeless beauty of care and understanding.

Avoid Idealization

The perception of reality is an active construction, where imagination, fantasy, and desire, of which romantic idealization is a figure, intervenes to transfigure reality.

From this point of view, we deduce that objectivity is an impossible ideal, and indeed it is.

The belief in knowing others objectively is one of the many illusions created by passion to avoid disappointment.

Psychoanalysis reminds lovers who idealize their loved ones that Idealization is an infantile regression because it transfers that onto the loved one asense of uniqueness that, as children, we used to associate with our parents.

If the idealization of parents is useful to children because it creates trust, it is terribly dangerous when you fall in love, because ideals tarnish and tricks sooner or later.

They come to the surface.

Dangerous but inevitable.

We depend on others; therefore, we are led to build them in the most stable terms possible. Our desire for security and our thirst for passion pushes us in opposite directions.

The other person's adored characteristics may not be illusory at all, mind you therefore to "healthy realism.".

Idolatrous love is marked by an intense and sudden romantic feeling where a person idealizes their loved one, projecting adoration onto them as a supreme being. This often happens when an individual hasn't attained a high level of maturity. In this process, the person loses a sense of self and seeks fulfillment through the loved one, expecting them to provide love, light, and happiness. However, since adoration is unsustainable in the long run, disappointment becomes inevitable. To cope, the person may move on to another idealized figure, creating an endless cycle. Despite being seen as true and great love, idolatrous love can reveal underlying feelings of hunger and desperation. Occasionally, both individuals may engage in mutual idolatry, creating a dynamic that can resemble madness in extreme cases.

Loving yourself before loving someone else

Falling in love is one of the most extraordinary and powerful feelings that a human being can experience. It's that magical moment when two people are attracted to each other, creating a deep connection and emotional bond. However, before you can truly love someone else, it is essential to fall in love with yourself and your life. In this article, we will explore the concept of falling in love before you can love someone else, based on studies and research in the fields of relationships and psychology.

The Importance of Self-Love

Self-love is the foundation of any healthy relationship and is essential to a person's emotional and mental well-being. Before you can share love with someone else, it is crucial to accept, appreciate, and respect yourself for who you are. A study published in the journal "Personality and Social Psychology Bulletin" highlighted that a high level of self-esteem is associated with more satisfying and long-lasting relationships.

Self-love does not mean being selfish or narcissistic, but rather recognizing your own value and authenticity. It involves the ability to take care of your own needs, develop healthy self-esteem, and accept your shortcomings.

Self-love includes several important aspects:

Self-Acceptance:

Accepting who you are, with all your strengths and weaknesses, is the first step towards falling in love with yourself. This means recognizing and embracing your imperfections without judgment.

Self-Care:

Taking care of your body and mind is an act of love for yourself. This includes good nutrition, exercise, rest, and maintaining balanced mental health.

Self-Respect:

Self-respect involves the ability to establish healthy boundaries in relationships and not allow others to treat us in a disrespectful or harmful manner.

Self-esteem:

High self-esteem is confidence in yourself and your abilities. It is the belief that you are worthy of love and happiness.

Independent Happiness:

Being happy with yourself and your life, regardless of a relationship, is a sign of self-love. We should not seek our happiness solely in romantic relationships.

Self-love and romantic relationships

When we fall in love with ourselves and take charge of our happiness, we are better able to establish healthy, balanced romantic relationships. Research published in the journal "Psychological Science" has shown that people with a high level of self-esteem tend to choose more compatible partners and maintain more positive relationships.

Additionally, when we truly love ourselves, we are more open to love and connection with others. We don't bring unresolved emotional baggage into relationships, which makes it easier to develop deep, authentic connections with our partners.

The Importance of Individual Wellbeing

Falling in love with oneself and one's life is closely linked to individual well-being. When we are happy and fulfilled individually, we are more attractive to others and more capable of building successful relationships. A study conducted by Harvard University found that personal well-being is a strong indicator of happiness in relationships.

How to cultivate self-love

Cultivating self-love takes time and effort, but it can lead to positive changes in your life and relationships. Here are some strategies for falling in love with yourself:

- Practice Gratitude: Take time each day to reflect on what you are grateful for in your life. This helps develop a positive outlook.

- Meditation and Mindfulness: Meditation and mindfulness can help you connect with yourself, reduce stress, and develop greater awareness.

- Self-curiosity: Be curious about yourself and your emotions. Find out what makes you happy, sad, or angry.

- Learn to forgive: Forgive yourself for past mistakes and don't hold grudges. Forgiveness is an act of self-love.

- Acceptance: Accept your flaws and imperfections. Nobody is perfect, and imperfections are what make us unique.

- Personal Growth: Commit to personal growth and achieving your goals. Making your dreams come true can boost your self-esteem.

Falling in love with yourself and your life is the first step towards creating healthy, meaningful romantic relationships. Self-love includes self-acceptance, self-care, self-respect, self-esteem, and independent happiness.

The Inner Child

The "inner child" is a term used to describe the emotional and psychological aspects of a person's character that retain memories, emotions, and experiences from their childhood. It symbolizes the childlike part within each individual, carrying with it the feelings and beliefs formed during early life. The idea is that these childhood experiences continue to shape how a person behaves, forms relationships, and responds emotionally as they grow older.

In therapy, the concept of the inner child is often explored to understand and address past emotional wounds, traumas, or unresolved issues from childhood. The aim is to integrate this inner child into the adult self, promoting emotional healing, self-awareness, and personal development. Various therapeutic approaches, including inner child therapy and inner child work, utilize this concept to help individuals navigate and heal from their past experiences.

Helping the inner child become a part of one's healing journey is a therapy process that deals with old emotional hurts from childhood. The inner child is like the younger version of a person, impacting how they think and act now. Therapists assist individuals in recognizing and understanding this inner child, creating a safe space to revisit childhood memories and emotions. Techniques like art or role-playing can help express these feelings.

Reparenting involves offering the care and support that might have been missing during childhood. The aim is to mend emotional wounds and use those lessons for positive changes in current life. Regular self-care is encouraged for ongoing support of the inner child. Usually, a trained therapist guides this transformative process.

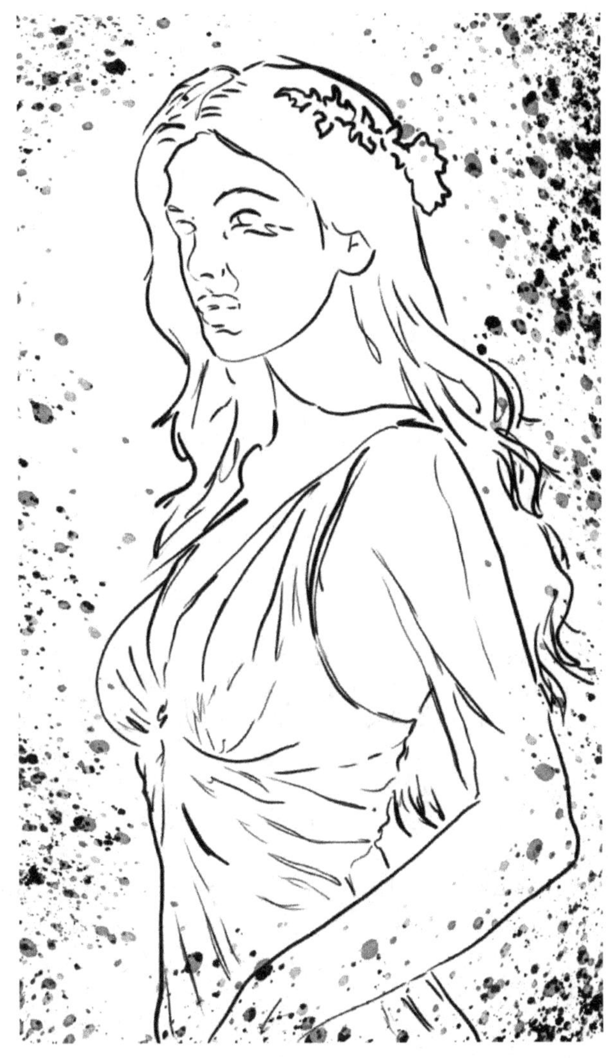

Self love

Cultivating self-love takes time, but lead to a fulfilling life and satisfying relationships. Before you can fully love someone else, you must fall in love with yourself.

5 LOVE LANGUAGE

Love uses words to give expression to what logic cannot grasp. In fact, love language paradoxes try to break it because logic includes normality and everyday life, while love wants to express the excess, the unusual, and cannot do so if it respects the rules of reasonableness. This excess grants love the freedom it needs because it arises when it is all-encompassing, and in fact, the language of excess demands totality, where hate and love can converge and pass through one another.

Communication is key. Eric Fromm, one of the biggest maestros of love, stressed the need for expressive communication. Learn the language of love, both verbal and non-verbal, to convey your feelings with finesse.

Presence

In a world consumed by distractions, genuine presence becomes an extraordinary gift, a magnetic force that draws hearts closer.

It's not just about being physically there; it's about cultivating a state of attentive awareness that transcends the superficial layers of interaction.

The art of listening

At the heart of presence lies the art of listening. It's not merely waiting for your turn to speak but immersing yourself in the melody of the other person's words.

Listening is an act of respect, an acknowledgment of the other's existence. It's a dance where words intertwine, creating a connection that transcends the mundane. In the realm of seduction, being an attentive listener is akin to composing a ballad that resonates in the corridors of the heart.

Eyes that speak

Your eyes, they say, are the windows to your soul. Fromm encourages us to harness the silent language of eye contact, a potent force in the art of presence. It's not a mere gaze; it's an unspoken dialogue, a dance of emotions that bypasses verbal barriers.

When your eyes meet, it's a moment of vulnerability and revelation. It's the acknowledgment of a shared existence that surpasses spoken language. In seduction, the power of your gaze becomes a silent vow, an unspoken promise of connection and understanding.

Genuine Interest

Presence is not a passive state but an active engagement, fueled by genuine interest. Fromm's wisdom encourages us to be curious and to explore the vast landscapes of the other person's thoughts and emotions. The authenticity of your interest becomes a radiant aura, drawing others into the warmth of your attention.

Ask questions not as a mere formality but as a genuine desire to unravel the layers of the other's being. Your interest becomes a beacon, guiding the way into the depths of connection. In the tapestry of seduction, curiosity is the brushstroke that paints vivid hues of fascination.

Physical Presence

Fromm's teachings extend beyond the realms of verbal communication, embracing the language of touch. Physical presence becomes an alchemical language of its own, capable of conveying emotions that words might falter to express.

A gentle touch, a reassuring hand on the shoulder—these gestures transcend the boundaries of spoken language. In the dance of seduction, physical presence becomes a silent conversation—an intimate dialogue that speaks volumes without uttering a single word.

In the realm of love, Erich Fromm beckons us to wield the power of presence as our most potent seductive tool. It's the symphony of listening, the dance of eye contact, the aura of genuine interest, and the silent language of touch that compose this masterpiece. As you navigate the landscapes of connection, remember: your presence is not just about being there; it's about creating a space where love and seduction intertwine in harmonious resonance.

Beyond Possession

Passion, when it doesn't lead to identification with the loved one, directs towards possession, which reduces the relationships of the loved one, and in which the lover doesn't really love his partner, but only the power he exercises over the other. So, the lover is not satisfied with the possession of the body and the sexual enjoyment of it derives, but demands that the loved one leave his entire world for him and that he loves him not only for his obvious identity but for his hidden qualities.

Only at this point his desire for possession is satisfied, but, with his satisfaction, so is his Passion is extinguished because it was not love for the other, but perverse self-love.

It is an intimacy that feeds on the deprivation of the world, because only through the exclusion of any relationship, the lover satisfies his desire for possession, which makes him feel unique, love has never granted itself.

Here jealousy, which is not a clue for genuine care , a sign of love, but a sign of the exclusivist conception of love.

This kind of relation that deprives the loved one of the enjoyment of the world, "the selfishness of two" regulated by one arises fusion without reciprocity where the desire for domination of one is combined with the desire for submission of the other.

There is also refugee possession. And since fear is stronger than desire, the world is stronger.

It's scary; the more the loved one becomes, that shelter that cannot be ignored.

It is about that imprisonment where the lover discovers that his sovereignty does not shine.

In substance, not only because its destiny is to be in the hands of others, but also through possession. But if the lover has no power over the world except for concession of the beloved, the possession that the lover intends to achieve over the beloved, it betrays all its radical and obstructive impotence.

A power of creation

Language empowers us to shape new realities, granting immense influence that can be harnessed positively, turning us into creators of a just society. Conversely, it can be wielded negatively, turning us into the creators of an unjust society marked by human and environmental violence and oppression. In our discussion on page 47, we labeled these as the soul's language and the ego's language. The former leads to the well-being of the soul and body, while the latter contributes to distress and illness.

Soul-sickness manifests in attention, perception, and memory disorders, prevalent across various societal levels. An attention deficit, for instance, signifies a disruption in voluntarily selecting the focus of our attention. This implies an inability to direct our attention to what we desire, causing distractions from what truly matters. In essence, our self-governance loses attentional sovereignty, hindering the essential task of focusing on elements crucial to happiness.

Losing attentional sovereignty extends to perceptual and mnemonic domains, ultimately affecting emotional sovereignty. Perceptual sovereignty diminishes as we no longer voluntarily choose what to perceive. Mnesic sovereignty weakens as we lose control over selecting memories. Consequently, unwanted perceptions and memories infiltrate, unimpeded by our psychic defenses, unable to differentiate between beneficial and detrimental elements.

The loss of thought sovereignty leads to a subsequent loss of emotional sovereignty—the ability to consciously evoke emotions that bring happiness while restraining those that induce unhappiness.

In the realm of self-governance, the ego possesses the ability to gain mastery over its adverse emotions and fully embrace the positive ones. This transformative shift occurs as the ego establishes a connection with its own soul or inner guide (daimon), which serves as the wellspring of heightened intelligence and creativity. Conversely, when negative emotions like anger, fear, or sadness take control of the ego, it succumbs to a state termed "captivus," essentially becoming a captive to these overpowering emotions.

Dependency replaces sovereignty, forcing a choice between autonomy and reliance on external sources of authority. The pivotal question arises: upon whom do we depend? Who exerts dominance and sovereignty over us?

Loneliness

The arousal of sexual desire can stem from various sources, such as the anxiety of solitude, the desire for conquest or submission, vanity, the wish to inflict harm, and even the intent to destroy. Love, too, has the power to evoke sexual desire, resulting in a physical connection marked by tenderness rather than lust or a conquest mentality. When the desire for physical union lacks the influence of love, and erotic love doesn't encompass fraternal love, it tends to lead to a superficial and illusory sense of fusion. Although sexual attraction may create a temporary illusion of union, the absence of love leaves individuals as estranged and divided as before, sometimes even fostering feelings of shame and hatred towards each other once the illusion fades. Tenderness, in Freud's view, is a sublimation of the sexual instinct and is a direct outcome of brotherly love, manifesting in both psychological and physical forms of affection.

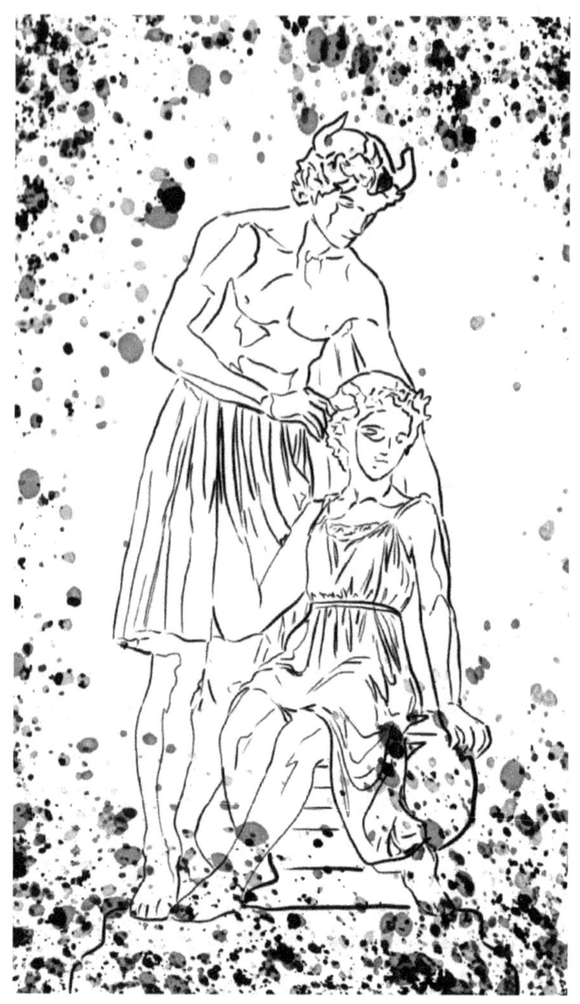

Love language

Love is an act of genuine presence and caring, not
selfish and egoistic fulfillment of personal self-love
who drives into possession and imprisonment.

6 BONDS

In these terms we can say that true love is moving from the conception of "I" to one of us, from love for the self as an individual to love for the entire unity of which the individual is part, and whose role and function is finally recognized as useful for the entire organism of which the "cell" is part, so love for the other is actually a projection of the resultant bonds that affect both the two cells involved, which from that bond will undergo transformations that both cells will evaluate as positive ... love for the other therefore becomes love for "us", and by projection, love for the entire organism of which that bond is inevitably part, which transfers its characteristic to the bonds with all the other cells.

It is not wrong to say that the type of bond we have with a person transfers all his characteristics by compensation to the others with which he is in contact.

Odi et Amo

In this new awareness, we understand that the very concept of an act of love for oneself, which provides for an inevitable perpetual transformation according to nature and involves effort and sacrifice, implies that the relationship with the loved one can also include pain, resulting from a mistake, a betrayal, a suffering, a wait, a disappointment, etc., from which those so-called "love pains" derive.

Love implies the acceptance and welcoming of every act of transformation that the relationship with the other brings to our being, without the claim that this is all just pleasant and enjoyable. Love is not pleasure or enjoyment; they are not concepts similar; rather, we could say that **true love is**, in this new light, actually **a love/hate relationship**, sharing of joy and suffering, of the totality of emotional nuances that a relationship entails.

JEALOUSY

To get control over this powerful state of mind, one must separate progressively love from obsessiveness, that is, civilize it.

Rational arguments always come after emotional ones.

Childhood evolution has more or less marked repercussions in adulthood, where exclusive love for the parent of the opposite sex is relived every time it is feared losing love for the person on whom you emotionally depend.

The echo of past experiences resonates with jealousy. Betrayal revives, in those who betray, the self-confidence and reactivates infantile narcissism. This is often the case in betrayals.

Narcissistic justification:

It is a torment or jealousy that alters perception, attention, memory, thoughts and behaviors.

Thought undergoes a real upheaval in its whirling around, amidst the idea of betrayal, to the point of touching the threshold of paranoid delirium, where even the more innocent and insignificant events are taken as irrefutable evidence than one's own.

Jealousy is absolutely justified.

Males tend to express their obsession by putting the problem on the table, tackling their rival and attacking their partner.

Female reactions tend more towards the internalization of pain with experiences of depression, insecurity and self-blame.

BETRAYAL

Betrayal lies in the original trust, where there is not even a trace of suspicion because neither the question nor the doubt arise. You don't give love without the possibility of a betrayal, just as there is no betrayal if you are not in a love relationship.

But the discovery of doubt marks the birth of consciousness, and this act is indicated by the betrayal.

The creative stimulus present in betrayal bears fruit only if the betrayed individual is the one.

Take a step forward, giving yourself an explanation of what happened.

Embrace this , it is necessary that the traitor does not justify the action and does not try to mitigate it.

With rational explanations, because of all the offenses, it will be the most burning for the betrayed person.

There are different reactions to betrayal:

1) revenge, which does not emancipate the soul but it stiffens it;

2) denial, in which the individual who has suffered a disappointment attempts to deny it the value of the other;

3) cynicism, which makes us believe that love is always a disappointment;

4) the self-betrayal, which leads to betraying oneself and one's emotional experiences;

5) the choice paranoid, an attitude linked more to the sphere of power than to that of love.

It seems that the law of life is written more in the name of betrayal than in that of fidelity.

Love and hate

Hate is the inevitable companion of love, and the survival of this feeling

Love does not depend so much on the ability to avoid aggression, which is a reflection of state of danger in which the person he loves finds himself, as well as the ability to experience it and go beyond it.

In love, the individual can accept dependence on the loved one or, to redeem it, transform loving passion into aggressive passion, full of hate, where the final message is that you can't do without this person.

The Mask

According to corenergetics, a newborn is likened to the seed of a tree, a tiny radiant soul brimming with love, requiring love for its growth. When encountering non-traumatized parents who accept, recognize, support, and value the child, this seed of expanding energy, this little soul, flourishes in an environment most conducive to its healthy development. However, finding parents without significant ego traits is relatively uncommon, making the majority of children, during their formative years, undergo shocks, abrupt suffering, and traumas resulting from their parents' lack of love. Corenergetics collectively label these various traumas as "the wound."

When the expansive energy within the child's small soul encounters the wound, the initial reaction is contraction, a withdrawal into itself. In simpler terms, if the suffering becomes overwhelming, the child feels rejected by the external world and harbors a desire to withdraw from life. This initial experience forms the basis of the depressed subpersonality, marked emotionally by a blend of fear and sadness—fear of abandonment and sadness stemming from the loss of love.

Yet, a second reaction swiftly emerges: anger, an intense fury directed at the perceived injustice endured. The Greeks term this passion "nemesis" and view it as an instinctive, life-sustaining reaction. This emotional response serves as the foundation of the narcissistic subpersonality, referred to as the "lower self" in Corenergetics.

It is evident that when confronted with trauma, the child's psyche undergoes a division from the outset: fear and sadness prompt withdrawal, while anger and fury drive towards aggression. As the child matures, a third, more intricate structure emerges: the mask. The mask adeptly navigates and moderates the two primary forces in perpetual conflict: withdrawal and closure on one side and aggression and hostility on the other. True to its name, the mask is a facade, a cover concealing underlying experiences—asocial in the first case, antisocial in the second.

The root of all malice lies here. By nature, humans are born sociable, group-oriented, and community-centric—*Homo homini deus.* However, due to unresolved traumas from early childhood, they lay the groundwork for their antithesis: *Homo homini lupus,* a threat to themselves and others. The mask embodies a small twist of the ego: pretense, falsehood, duplicity, and concealment, constituting the fundamental traits of the ego.

The ego embodies an insoluble conflict, a realm of suffering, pathology, and an oscillation between asociality and antisociality.

Through the corenergetics model, we gain insight into the origin of subpersonalities—the traumas, abandonment, oppression, and injustice endured by the child by those meant to care for them. There exist at least ten primary subpersonalities, familiar to all: depressive, oral, masochistic, phobic, obsessive, paranoid, narcissistic, schizoid, histrionic, and psychosomatic. In traditional clinical practice and even in modern cognitive theories, these subpersonalities are often categorized, diagnosed, and treated as personality disorders. The danger lies in diagnoses transforming into labels, permanently affixed by the individual, such as "I am obsessive," "I am not, I am depressed." These statements reflect egoistic thought, causing harm to the person uttering or thinking them. The subpersonality model, when properly explained and understood, is less susceptible to this distorted use of language. We are not defined by our subpersonalities; rather, we are defined by our soul.

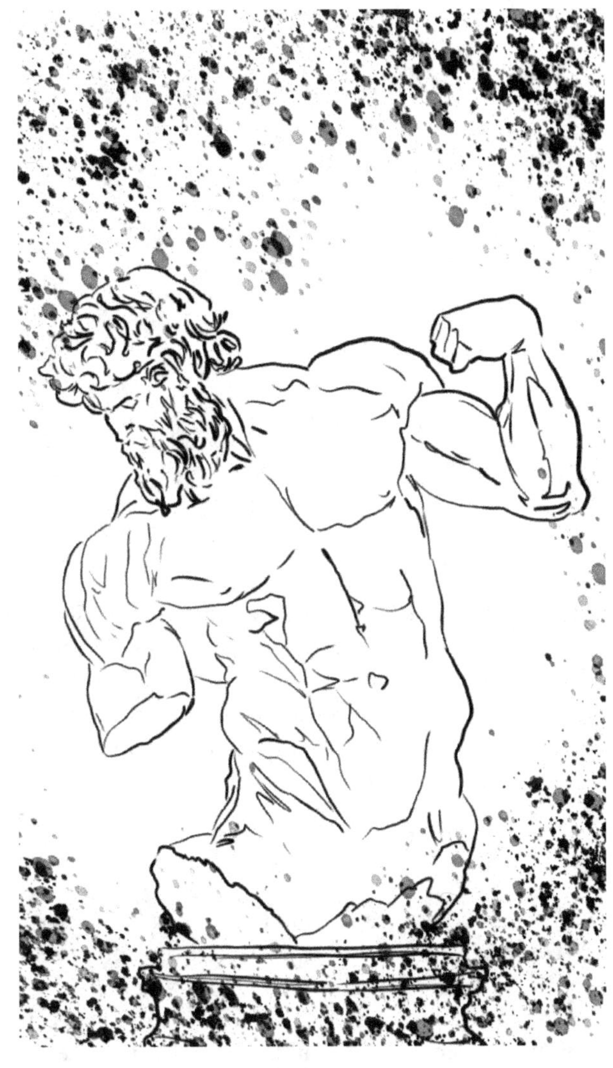

Bonds

Our bond with each other is actually a projection of
self, and in this light true love for the other is actually
a love for the entire unity of which we are a part.

7 SEDUCTION

One significant aspect of Freud's exploration of love is the concept of libido, which he defined as the psychic energy associated with life instincts. Libido, for Freud, is not solely sexual but encompasses a broader life force that influences various aspects of the human experience, including love.

Initially, Freud considered seduction to be a key factor in the development of neuroses, particularly during his early work with patients who reported early traumatic experiences, often involving sexual abuse. Freud theorized that repressed memories of childhood seduction events could lead to psychological distress and the manifestation of neurotic symptoms.

However, he later modified his stance during what is known as the "seduction theory controversy."

He eventually shifted his emphasis from actual childhood sexual abuse events to the idea of repressed fantasies and unconscious desires. Freud proposed that some patients' memories of seduction were not accurate representations of events but rather distorted recollections stemming from their own unconscious fantasies.

In the later stages of his work, Freud focused on his most famous relevant concept: the Oedipus complex, where he proposed that during early childhood, a child develops unconscious desires for his mother (his or her opposite-sex parent) and may experience rivalry with his father (the same-sex parent).

While not explicitly about seduction, this complex lays the foundation for later relationships and can contribute to a man's approach to intimate connections.

In the context of sexual inhibition with women one esteems, Freud might suggest that deep-seated psychological conflicts or anxieties, often rooted in the unconscious, play a role. For instance, the fear of disappointing or being judged by a woman one highly respects could create anxiety that interferes with sexual performance.

Freud also emphasized the role of societal norms and cultural expectations in shaping sexual behavior. The superego, a component of the psyche representing internalized societal values, could contribute to a man feeling inhibited when engaging sexually with a woman he holds in high regard.

Moreover, the concept of libido, representing the psychic energy associated with life instincts, comes into play.

The redirection of libido towards pursuits beyond sexual gratification, such as intellectual or creative endeavors, could be a manifestation of sublimation, a defense mechanism Freud theorized.

Freud's exploration of seduction initially centered on the impact of real traumatic events, but he later shifted toward understanding the role of unconscious fantasies and desires in shaping an individual's psychology. The concept of seduction in Freudian terms is closely tied to the broader framework of psychoanalytic theory, emphasizing the importance of unconscious motivations in human behavior.

Consider the seductive arts not as manipulation but as an invitation to connect, to enthrall, and to create an atmosphere charged with desire.

Mastering the seductive arts involves a combination of self-awareness, genuine connection, and a deep understanding of human psychology.

Here's a step-by-step guide:

LOVE AND SEDUCTION

In daily life, transparency manages to broaden the horizon and open up the scenario from the imagination. In fact, desire is found in every crack of reality that it leaves.

A further meaning shines through: that of the unreal and de-real. The other's body becomes as well a mirror reflecting our desire, and this body must never be naked, because seduction is expressed through clothes, accessories, gestures, and music.

LOVE AND PRODENCE

Love requires our ego to love and be loved, one of the two subjectivity present in every individual and which, against generic sexuality, imposes the barrier of modesty. However, it does not limit sexuality but identifies it, removing it from that genericity in which pleasure is celebrated without recognizing individuality. It's important emphasize that modesty is not an exclusively sexual feeling but also has a social value that aims to defend the individual against the advertising of private.

LOVE AND SOLITUDE

Greek mythology had deified masturbation because it was an expression of self-sufficiency and independence from others.

But this act was condemned, in the age of Enlightenment, from medical science and economics: The first maintained that it caused diseases, while the second stated that it was a waste. Instead, observing the phenomenon of masturbation from a different perspective from these two disciplines, this "vice of the adolescent" does not appear as something to fight.

LOVE AND MONEY

Prostitution is an exchange of sex and money that characterizes the sexual regime of our society, which is fueled by a desire for rapid improvement of own economic conditions. In fact, when faced with money, everything becomes a commodity.

When a man pays a woman, he does not recognize any interiority of his own, arriving at consider it more as a "genre" than as an "individual".

LOVE AND PASSION

Unlike love, passion does not follow the rules; it ignores self-government; it does not knows the limit and does not depend on projects. This is why it is possible to say that love is Christian, while passion is pagan.

Passion seeks reassurance, but in the same time wants to be proven wrong, rejected, and disappointed because it attributes affection to domesticity, loving, and being loved have little importance, because passion knows destiny and not exchange, as the other is considered only a matter for his creation, that is, fantasy, which feeds on doubt and uncertainty.

It is possible to say that love is Christian and the passion is pagan. Passion transfigures and the material it feeds on is imagination.

Passion can continue its creative process only if it is fueled by the doubt and uncertainty that keep the child awake desire, and long live the spark.

Let's discuss now the psychological aspects of seduction, emphasizing that it extends beyond physical attraction. Individuals can be seduced mentally, emotionally, and spiritually by various factors, including societal norms, ideologies, and personal desires.

Conscious and unconscious seduction

We need to distinguish between conscious and unconscious seduction. Unconscious seduction involves individuals being influenced by societal expectations, norms, and cultural ideals without full awareness. Conscious seduction, on the other hand, implies intentional efforts to influence others, whether positively or negatively.

The Seduction of Consumer Culture

Modern society faces the seductive nature of consumer culture, where individuals are enticed by materialism, superficial values, and the pursuit of wealth.

People can be seduced into conforming to societal norms that may not align with genuine human needs for connection and meaning.

Seduction in Relationships

Individuals can be seduced within the context of intimate relationships. This involves the complexities of attraction, the dynamics of power, and the role of love. A deeper understanding of oneself and others leads to navigating the seductive elements within relationships.

Self-Seduction

Embrace the role of self-awareness in resisting negative seductions and cultivating a healthy sense of self. He encourages individuals to be conscious of their desires, motivations, and the influences that shape their values. By understanding oneself, one can resist being seduced into conformity that goes against authentic needs.

Freedom and Responsibility

Seduction is intertwined with the notions of freedom and responsibility; individuals can resist negative seductions and live authentically by exercising their freedom to choose and taking responsibility for their choices.

Love as an Antidote to Negative Seduction

Love, understood as an active and ongoing process rather than a passive feeling, is an antidote to negative seductions. Genuine love involves a deep connection, mutual understanding, and a commitment to the well-being of oneself and others.

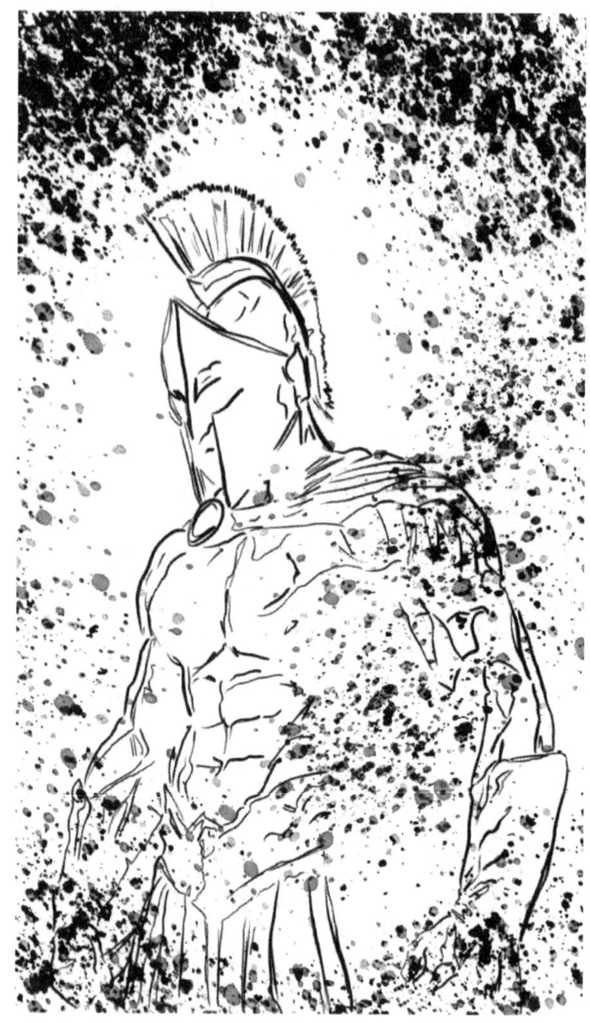

Seduction

Mastering the seductive arts is not about manipulation , but fostering genuine connections, appreciating the uniqueness of each individual.

8 INTIMACY

Giving

In love, the art of giving transcends mere material offerings. It involves the selfless sharing of time, attention, and emotional support.

Giving in love is a profound expression of care, demonstrating a commitment to the well-being and happiness of others. It's not confined to grand gestures; even the smallest acts of kindness can create a lasting impact. The art lies in understanding the unique needs and desires of your partner and offering support without expectation of reciprocation. True giving involves listening, empathy, and a willingness to contribute to the growth and joy of the relationship. It transforms love from a passive state to an active, nurturing force, fostering a connection that deepens with each shared moment and thoughtful gesture. The art of giving in love is a continual dance of generosity, enriching the bond between partners and creating a harmonious symphony of mutual care and appreciation.

Intimacy with unconscius

According to Freudian theory, intimacy is deeply connected to the unconscious mind and the interplay of complex psychological forces.

Freud proposed that the unconscious mind serves as a reservoir of desires, including those of a sexual and intimate nature. Within this reservoir, he identified the id as the primal, instinctual force seeking immediate gratification of desires. The ego, on the other hand, functions as the conscious mediator, navigating between the demands of the id, societal norms, and reality.

Finally, the superego represents internalized societal values and moral standards.

In the context of love and intimacy, Freud argued that individuals are driven by unconscious desires and fantasies that shape their romantic pursuits. He introduced the concept of eros, the life instinct, which includes the drive for love, creativity, and connection. The unconscious, according to Freud, plays a pivotal role in shaping one's attractions and forming the basis for intimate connections.

Freud's exploration of intimacy in love emphasizes the importance of acknowledging and understanding the unconscious forces that influence human relationships.

Mistery

Freud's concept of the unconscious mind accentuates the enchantment of mystery in human relationships. According to Freudian theory, the unconscious harbors hidden desires, motivations, and fantasies that shape our behaviors, including those within the realm of love. Freud suggests that the unconscious is not readily accessible to conscious awareness, creating an element of mystery in understanding one's own desires and the motives driving interpersonal connections.

The allure of mystery, as proposed by Freud, lies in the gradual unfolding of the unconscious. By not revealing everything at once, the unconscious becomes a reservoir of intrigue and fascination. This deliberate unveiling keeps the flames of desire burning, fostering a dynamic and enduring sense of attraction. In Freudian terms, the unconscious adds depth to human connections, making love a journey of discovery where the enigmatic nature of desires and emotions continually captivates, ensuring that the allure of the mysterious remains an integral part of the tapestry of love.

Vulnerability

In the exploration of human connection, we embrace vulnerability as a catalyst for authentic intimacy. True connection necessitates openness and honesty, encouraging individuals to lay bare their authentic selves.

By shedding the protective layers, one creates a path to genuine intimacy, where the raw and unfiltered aspects of one's being can resonate with another.

Vulnerability is not a weakness but a courageous act of revealing one's true essence. In exposing our genuine selves, we invite reciprocity and deepen the bonds of understanding. This vulnerability becomes the cornerstone of authentic relationships, fostering an environment where trust, empathy, and true connection can flourish.

Commitment

Our society is characterized by individualism, in which the individual lives according to his own personal idea of happiness without being influenced by traditional norms.

Currently, Love is disconnected from any social, legal, or religious reference and is spreading the figure of "the man of passion," who awaits some revelation about himself from love or about life in general.

On the one hand, therefore, love-passion, which represents escape from the world to reach absolute happiness in a dream; on the other hand, the love action that establishes marriage, which does not escape from the world but assumes its commitment to it, where, we could say, the absolutizing romantic element leaves room for the dedication to the well-being of the partner and respect for shared values.

Intimacy plays a crucial role in the art of seduction, enriching the depth and authenticity of the connection between individuals. While seduction is often associated with the initial stages of attraction, intimacy takes the interaction to a more profound and meaningful level.

Emotional Connection:

Intimacy fosters a strong emotional connection between individuals. Beyond physical attraction, sharing emotions, thoughts, and vulnerabilities creates a bond that goes beyond the surface level, contributing to a more profound and genuine connection.

Trust and vulnerability:

Intimacy requires a level of trust and the willingness to be vulnerable. When individuals feel secure enough to open up to each other, it creates a sense of closeness and authenticity that enhances the seductive experience.

Understanding Desires:

Intimacy allows individuals to understand each other's desires on a deeper level. This understanding goes beyond the superficial and helps tailor the seductive interaction to align with each person's unique preferences and needs.

Mindful Presence:

Intimacy encourages mindful presence during the seductive process. Being fully engaged and attuned to the other person's thoughts, feelings, and cues enhances the overall experience and demonstrates a genuine interest in the connection.

Communication of Intentions:

Through intimacy, individuals can communicate their intentions more effectively. This involves expressing desires, boundaries, and expectations, fostering clear and respectful communication that enriches the seductive exchange.

Shared Experiences:

Intimacy often involves sharing experiences, whether they are personal stories, dreams, or mutual interests. Shared experiences create a sense of unity and connection, enhancing the seductive journey by building a foundation of common ground.

Long-Term Attraction:

While the initial stages of seduction may focus on physical attraction, intimacy contributes to a sustainable and long-term connection. A relationship built on intimacy is more likely to endure and deepen over time, extending the allure beyond the initial seductive encounter.

Mutual Enjoyment:

Intimacy ensures that the seductive experience is mutually enjoyable. By understanding each other's preferences and boundaries, individuals can create an environment where both parties feel comfortable, valued, and respected.

Depth of Understanding:

Intimacy allows for a deeper understanding of the other person's values, beliefs, and aspirations. This knowledge contributes to a more nuanced and meaningful seductive interaction, fostering a connection that transcends the surface level.

Fulfillment of Emotional Needs:

Intimacy addresses emotional needs, providing a sense of fulfillment that goes beyond the physical realm. When individuals feel emotionally connected and understood, the seductive experience becomes more gratifying and satisfying.

Just as emotional intelligence involves recognizing, understanding, and managing emotions, intimacy requires recognizing, understanding, and navigating the emotional connections between individuals. Both emotional intelligence and intimacy entail skills such as self-awareness, regulation of emotions, motivation, empathy, and effective interpersonal communication. Just as emotional intelligence enhances personal and professional success, intimacy fosters deeper and more meaningful connections in personal relationships. Individuals with high emotional intelligence and a capacity for intimacy can navigate emotional complexities, build strong relationships, and foster positive interactions in various aspects of life.

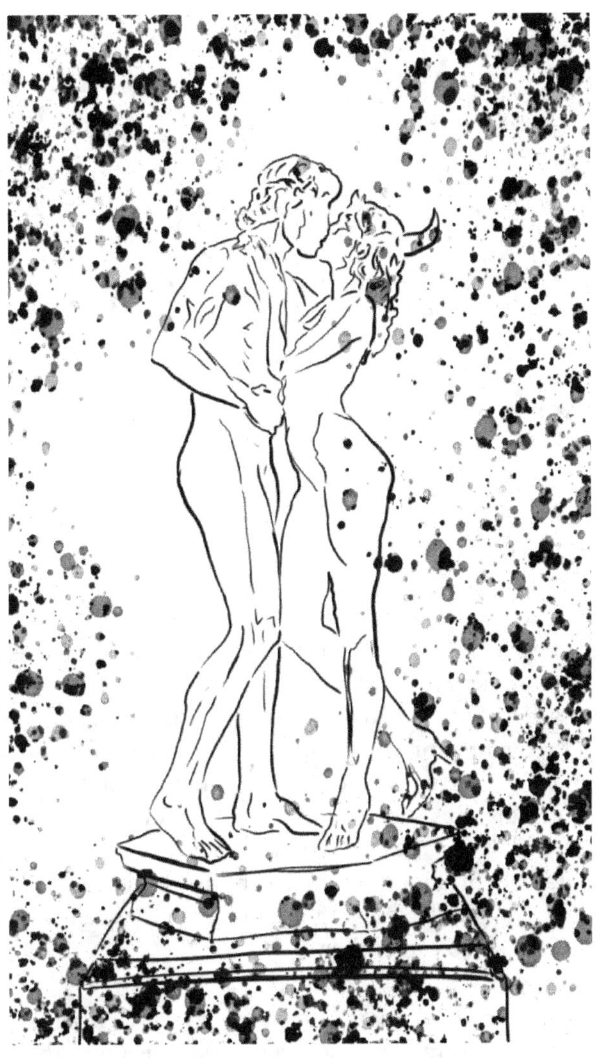

Intimacy

Intimacy goes beyond the external allure and
contributes to a more profound and meaningful
exchange between individuals.

9 CONTACT

Erotic love, unlike brotherly or maternal love, is characterized by the merging of two distinct individuals into a unified entity. It tends to be exclusive rather than universal, making it one of the most misleading forms of love. Frequently mistaken for the initial stages of "falling in love," where barriers between strangers crumble unexpectedly, this sense of sudden intimacy is inherently short-lived. Once the initial barriers are dismantled and the beloved becomes intimately known, the illusion of true understanding fades, leaving the individuals equally known and unknown to each other.

In erotic love, intimacy is often equated with sexual contact. Overcoming physical separation becomes the focal point, as the sense of being apart is primarily experienced on a physical level. The quest for refuge from solitude finds solace in this form of love, creating a mutual alliance against the world. However, this alliance, though labeled as love and intimacy, often carries a subtle undertone of two-way selfishness.

Building a profound sexual connection involves open communication, emotional intimacy, trust, and mutual respect. Both partners should be present in the moment, exploring each other's desires, and maintaining variety and novelty. Shared goals, physical touch, and self-awareness contribute to a deep connection that goes beyond the physical realm. Foster a sense of security and reliability, and be open to exploring new aspects of intimacy together. Prioritize the emotional and physical well-being of both partners for a fulfilling and lasting connection.

Touch

In its intricate exploration of human connection, "Sensual Symbiosis" delves into the realm of touch and sensuality, drawing inspiration from Freud's concept of pleasure-seeking behavior. At the heart of this chapter lies the mastery of the art of touch—an art that transcends the physical and reaches into the realms of emotion and desire.

Freud's insights into pleasure-seeking behavior become a crucial guide, emphasizing the profound impact of tactile experiences on human connection. The chapter advocates for the artful navigation of touch, where it goes beyond the surface to create a symbiotic connection. This connection, when mastered, possesses the captivating power to intertwine two individuals in a dance of shared pleasure and profound intimacy.

"Sensual Symbiosis" invites readers to recognize touch as a language of its own, a conduit for expressing desire, care, and emotional resonance. By understanding the intricacies of pleasure-seeking behavior, individuals can harness the transformative potential of touch, creating a symbiotic connection that transcends the physical and weaves an intricate tapestry of profound and captivating intimacy.

Balance

In the exploration of relationships, "Balancing Power" draws wisdom from Freud's insights on power dynamics. Freud emphasized the delicate equilibrium required in relationships, steering clear of dominance or submission. This chapter advocates for the art of finding balance—a key element in fostering mutual respect and sustaining enduring desire.

Freud's observations on power dynamics underscore the importance of neither overpowering nor relinquishing control in relationships. Striking a harmonious balance ensures a partnership where both individuals contribute to the relationship's dynamics without suppressing each other. This equilibrium becomes the foundation for a relationship built on shared decision-making, cooperation, and respect.

"Bridging Power" guides readers to navigate the intricacies of power dynamics, promoting an environment where neither partner holds excessive sway. Instead, it encourages the cultivation of a relationship where power is shared, allowing both individuals to thrive while preserving the allure of desire. By embracing balance, couples can forge a lasting connection founded on equality, ensuring that power dynamics contribute positively to the vibrancy and resilience of their shared journey.

Vision

This chapter guides readers in the creation of a personalized "Love Manifesto." Drawing inspiration from Freud's pleasure-seeking behavior concept, it encourages individuals to articulate their unique vision of love. By crafting a manifesto, readers delve into their desires, expectations, and values within relationships. The process involves introspection and thoughtful consideration, aligning personal beliefs with the pursuit of genuine connection. By manifesting their ideals, individuals gain clarity on the elements vital to their happiness in love, steering their romantic journey with intention and purpose. "Crafting Your Love Manifesto" serves as a compass, helping readers navigate the complexities of relationships while embracing the individuality and authenticity that form the foundation of their personal love narrative.

Consider sharing examples or anecdotes to illustrate the impact of a love manifesto. Highlight stories of individuals who, through the intentional creation of their guiding principles in love, found clarity, fulfillment, and authentic connections. This approach adds relatability and authenticity, demonstrating that the crafting of a love manifesto is a practical and empowering step in one's romantic journey.

In summary, crafting your love manifesto is not just a literary exercise but a powerful act of intention—a declaration that shapes the trajectory of your romantic endeavors.

Orgasm

Sacredness is due to man's desire for immortality and therefore to the desire for preserve the survival of the individual and of the totality of being.

The totality of being has nothing to do with death;

Actually, death of the individual manifests it with his eternity.

In addition to sacrifice, another way to experience the death of one's individuality is orgasm, the pinnacle of sexual life, during which the I and the You dissolve, and this is made possible by mutual trust.

Trust guarantees a return.

On the one hand, we can hardly tolerate the condition that binds us to individuality; on the other hand, we cannot

We are immune to nostalgia.

The ban, which, however, remains in place, protects us from this nostalgia; break by transgression.

Just like homicidal violence, sexual relations are prohibited within archaic societies.

In fact, not only is death beyond measure for the single individual, but also birth is beyond measure; arises from sexuality and brings with it a sense of excess.

If it is part of man's nature to be able to survive, it is evident that everything that threatens, this possibility appears to be unnatural.

Love is sacred as a transgressive activity that opposes prohibition, whatever it is; Notable in the sexual prohibition is its full revelation of transgression.

Joy and Sadness

People often say that happiness arises when we find something or someone pleasing. Numerous words can better convey this emotional state by accentuating various aspects. For instance, we may express feeling "fascinated" or even "in love" when drawn to a person—the former often linked to their abilities or attitudes, and the latter when the source of our strong emotions isn't immediately identifiable. Joy may accompany our time with a person we like, leading us to articulate feeling "enjoyed" because we find it entertaining. Alternatively, we might say we feel "passionate" when pleasure is associated with both a person and an activity we particularly enjoy. Another way to express satisfaction, with a focus on fulfilling a need, is to say we feel "satisfied." This heightened satisfaction can induce a sense of fullness, temporarily diverting us from a quest or motivating us to maintain the gratifying situation.

These emotions contribute to the cultivation of positive self-esteem, seeking to foster a healthy relationship with oneself.

It's frequently mentioned that we experience sadness when an event jeopardizes our connection with someone significant, whether it's a romantic partner, spouse, parent, friend, or relative. Numerous words exist that can more precisely convey this emotional state by highlighting different facets.

For instance, we might say that we feel "sorry" if we've done something that causes the other person distress or if the other person's actions or words have hurt us. Another term, "disappointed," carries even more intensity, especially when we had specific expectations about someone or ourselves that didn't materialize. For example, if I anticipate my child excelling at school and he instead brings home poor grades, the prevalent emotion is often one of disappointment.

However, when someone we love fails to acknowledge us, disregards us, or even despises certain aspects of our character, we may experience the emotion of feeling "rejected." In a group context, the term "excluded" comes into play—applicable when friends omit us from an invitation or when family alliances sideline a member.

Sadness can also manifest when we find ourselves in the company of someone incompatible with or seemingly distant from our sensibilities, leading us to express feeling "bored." It's essential to note that defining a visibly sad person as "depressed" is a common misconception.

Depression is a genuine pathology where the emotion of sadness persists, not tied to a specific situation but due to an ongoing medical condition.

Misconceptions about love often lead people to believe it should be devoid of conflict. In reality, many conflicts are attempts to evade genuine issues. True conflicts, however, are not destructive; they lead to clarification and personal growth. Love thrives when individuals communicate from their deepest selves, forming the foundation for genuine connection. Harmony or conflict becomes secondary to the profound reality of being true to oneself. The depth of relationships and the vitality of each individual signify the presence of true love.

Scheduled Sex

In theme of sexual education within the context of sustaining a long-term marriage, a recent trend among sexologists and theorists is to prioritize the sexual aspect as a cornerstone for a fulfilling relationship. Expanding on this notion, some propose likening it to a sport or hobby, advocating for its inclusion in daily routines akin to a work commitment. However, while this approach may seem pragmatic on paper, it fundamentally undermines the essence of genuine love and the emotional underpinnings of sexual desire. In such a scenario, eros, the profound connection and passion between partners, risks being reduced to a mere mechanical act, devoid of evolution, intimacy, or genuine connection with the other person. Instead, it becomes a self-serving pursuit, where one indulges in the gratification of personal desires without regard for the deeper bond or mutual fulfillment within the relationship.

Love must embrace its inherent mystery, characterized by its unpredictability, where no strategy focused solely on ensuring the longevity of a relationship through sexual activity can truly provide assurance. Love is found in the raw experience of each moment, encompassing both its luminous and obscure facets and acknowledging both its fleetingness and its capacity for profound transformation. When expressed erotically, love transcends the structured and regimented approaches advocated by contemporary sexologists, instead embodying a rich tapestry of emotions and connections that defy rigid categorization.

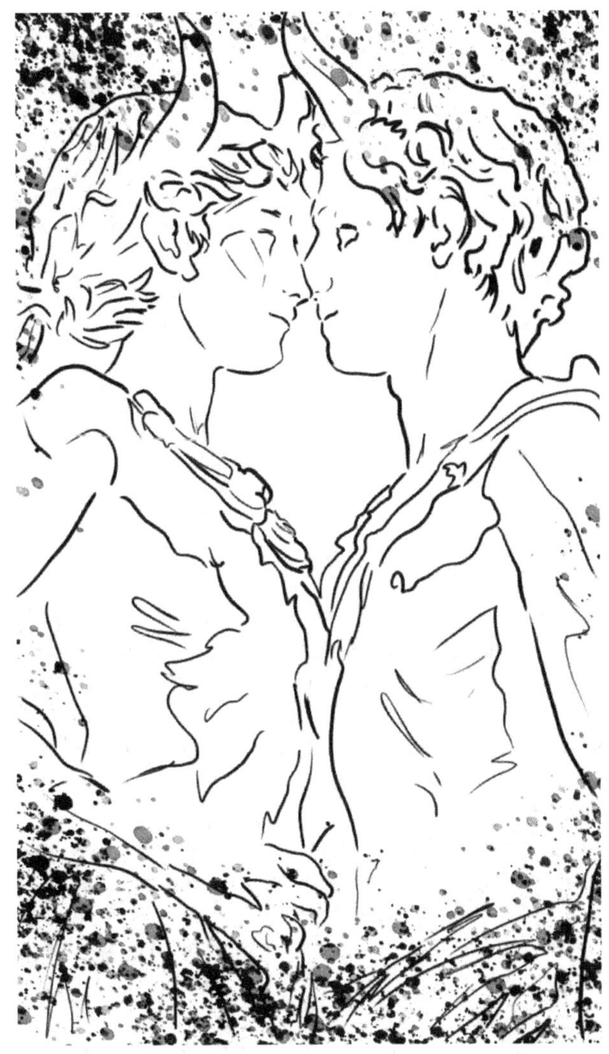

Contact

Immature love adheres to the principle: "I love because I am loved", while mature love operates on the principle: "I am loved cause I love."

10 SHADOW

Unfortunately, there is no doubt that human beings are generally less good than we imagine or desire; each of us carries with us a dark shadow of personality that the ego does not want to recognize. The shadow is a living part of the personality and therefore wishes to coexist with it in some way. We cannot deny its existence; we cannot use reason to free ourselves from it. The more the shadow is not integrated into the conscious life of the individual, the darker and more dense it becomes, becoming an unconscious obstacle that frustrates our good intentions until sooner or later a fracture occurs in the psychic system.

Facing this shadow is the first test of courage on the inner journey, a test sufficient to scare most people because the encounter with ourselves is one of the most unpleasant things, but if we are able to observe our own shadow and endure to know its contents, then a small part of the problem is already solved. At least we have brought the personal unconscious to light. The shadow is that part of the personality that we refuse to recognize because it contains all our negative qualities: destructive tendencies, perverse inclinations, aggressiveness, atrocities, lust, and brutality.

All those qualities and tendencies that do not harmonize with collective values—everything that avoids the light of public opinion—come together to form the shadow;

The shadow is a set of dark aspects that each of us, without exception, carries within ourselves but that are socially unacceptable. We repress them to prevent them from expressing themselves because we don't want others to know that there is a part of us capable of committing monstrous acts, and we don't even want others to know. We push all this into the basement, where it remains unknown; however, they do not disappear but function autonomously. Our shadow continues to operate from the unconscious, acting as a spirit that has possessed its own will and exercises control over our thoughts, emotions, and behaviors that tend to be mostly destructive and self-destructive.

This may be the reason why it is so difficult for us to get our lives in order, even if we know what is good for us and have committed to doing what is good for us or stopping doing what is harmful to us.

Our shadow cancels this conscious part and drags us into the same destructive inertia over and over again, as Robert Louis Stevenson indicates in his famous book "The Strange Case of Dr. Jackill and Mr. Hide." Man is not one but truly two.

He has a personality and a shadow, each fighting for supremacy in his mind.

To avoid being victims of shadow possession, we must become aware of those dark qualities that are buried in the unconscious and integrate them into our personalities.

No progress or growth is possible until the shadow is properly integrated. When you are not aware of your shadow, you declare that a part of your personality does not exist.

That part then enters the realm of the non-existent and magnifies, assuming enormous proportions, relegated to a projection of fear.

If you get rid of the qualities you don't like by denying them, you become more and more unconscious of who you are.

You declare yourself more and more non-existent, and your demons get fatter and fatter. Instead of labeling those aspects of ourselves as abominable, shadow integration requires that we begin to see them as necessary and vital parts of our being.

However, Carl Jung argues that this integration is extremely difficult, as most people will not admit that deep down they are not completely virtuous, selfless, and good human beings but instead contain destructive and immoral selfish impulses and capacities.

Most delude themselves by placing themselves on a pedestal of false goodness, thus continuing to be fragmented and incomplete individuals who project their own darkness onto others.

The encounter with oneself is, first of all, the encounter with one's own shadow; it is a narrow passage, a narrow door of painful constriction that no one can escape. It goes deep into the well, but you have to learn to know yourself to know who you really are. The potential to commit the most horrible acts is present in every human being, and this includes you too. The worst barbarities committed by other individuals throughout history are atrocities that you could end up committing, and we see proof of this daily with acts of people who apparently would never have committed violence and murder, yet they reach a point of no return. Why?

The most despicable part of the human condition lives within you, and repressing all of this only feeds the monster, which eventually takes control of your unconscious and makes your life a disaster.

What happens when you stop repressing the worst in you and integrate it harmoniously into your psychic structure?

The best of you begins to emerge because the shadow not only contains destructive aspects of the personality but also very powerful creative abilities that we repressed growing up.

The shadow reveals a number of good qualities, such as normal instincts, appropriate reactions, realistic intuitions, creative impulses, etc.

Many of the traits and impulses we have repressed have repressed much of our innate talents and abilities.

So when the shadow integrates, we achieve what I call individuation.

Individuation means becoming an individual. understanding individuality as our most internal, ultimate, and incomparable peculiarity.

Therefore, individuation could be translated as becoming oneself.

How do we integrate our shadow?

Carl Jung states that there is no universally effective technique for assimilating the shadow; it is more similar to either diplomacy or the art of government and is always an individual matter.

First of all, it is necessary to accept and take seriously the existence of the shadow. Second, it is necessary to become aware of one's own qualities and intentions; this happens through careful observation of our moods and fantasies. Thirdly, a long process of negotiation is inevitable: if the shadow is the gateway to our being, we must dare and descend into its infernal depths and face all the dark aspects of ourselves;

In myths, the hero is the one who defeats the dragon, not the one who is devoured by it; furthermore, the one who has never confronted the dragon or who, if he has, then claims not to have seen anything is not a hero. Similarly, only he who ventures to fight the dragon and is not defeated by it obtains the treasure; only he has a legitimate right to self-confidence because he has faced the dark territory of himself and earned himself.

This experience gives a little faith and trust in the ability of the self to support us since everything that threatened from within has been conquered and has acquired the right to believe that it will be able to overcome all future threats with its own internal means.

Individual into society

Love serves as a foundational and transformative force that shapes individuals, relationships, and communities. Here are several ways in which love contributes to the construction of a positive society:

Empathy and compassion:

Love fosters empathy and compassion, encouraging individuals to understand and care for the well-being of others. In a positive society, a collective sense of empathy creates a supportive environment where individuals look out for one another.

Community Building:

Love promotes a sense of community and belonging. When people genuinely care for each other, they are more likely to collaborate, support shared goals, and actively contribute to the well-being of the community.

Social Cohesion:

Love strengthens social bonds and promotes cohesion within a society. Positive interpersonal relationships, built on love and mutual respect, create a sense of unity that transcends differences and fosters harmonious coexistence.

Altruism and Philanthropy:

Love motivates altruistic actions and philanthropy. Individuals who have a deep sense of love for humanity are more likely to engage in charitable activities, contributing to the betterment of society as a whole.

Conflict Resolution:

Love encourages constructive approaches to conflict resolution. In a positive society, individuals are more likely to address conflicts with empathy, understanding, and a commitment to finding mutually beneficial solutions.

Education and Nurturing:

Love is fundamental to the upbringing and education of individuals. A society that values love prioritizes nurturing environments for children, emphasizing education that fosters emotional intelligence, empathy, and positive values.

Mental health and well-being:

Love contributes to the mental health and well-being of individuals. A society that prioritizes love and emotional support creates conditions for better mental health outcomes, reducing stress, loneliness, and mental health disparities.

Generosity and Sharing:

Love encourages generosity and the willingness to share resources. In a positive society, individuals are more likely to contribute to the common good by sharing resources, knowledge, and opportunities.

Cultural Enrichment:

Love for the arts, culture, and diversity enhances the richness of a society. A positive society values and celebrates its cultural diversity, fostering an environment where different perspectives are respected and embraced.

Environmental Stewardship:

Love extends to the natural world, promoting environmental stewardship. A society that values love for the environment is more likely to engage in sustainable practices, conservation efforts, and the protection of ecosystems for future generations.

Ethical Decision-Making:

Love influences ethical decision-making. In a positive society, individuals are guided by a sense of love for humanity, promoting ethical behavior and responsible decision-making in various aspects of life.

Resilience and Solidarity:

Love contributes to resilience and solidarity during challenging times. A society grounded in love is better equipped to navigate crises, support one another, and foster a sense of solidarity in the face of adversity.

In essence, love is a powerful force that shapes the values, behaviors, and interactions within a society. It creates a positive foundation that influences individual well-being and contributes to the collective flourishing of communities. Cultivating a culture of love fosters a society where kindness, empathy, and cooperation thrive, laying the groundwork for a positive and harmonious coexistence.

Evolution

In the final exploration, "The Eternal Flame" encapsulates the essence of love as an ever-evolving journey. Drawing insights from both Freud and Fromm, this chapter imparts the wisdom to learn, adapt, and nurture the flame of love. The art of love, as illuminated by these masters, is a perpetual process of growth and connection-building, resilient against the passage of time.

This chapter underscores that love, enriched by the teachings of Freud and Fromm, is not a static but a dynamic force requiring continuous adaptation and learning. By assimilating the wisdom of these perspectives, individuals can stoke the eternal flame of their relationships. The artistry of love lies in the commitment to evolving together, weathering challenges, and constructing a connection that endures the trials of time. "The Eternal Flame" serves as a poignant reminder that, in the grand tapestry of love, the journey is never truly complete but rather an ongoing expedition of shared experiences, growth, and the perpetual renewal of the flame that kindles enduring connection.

God

The metaphor of God has always been connected to the
metaphor of love, in the sense that without the presence of
transcendence, that is, that which is beyond the limits of all
possible knowledge and therefore superior to human
reason, love loses its strength and its ability to read the
world.

An enigma remains where love sees its transcendence in
God, and God sees its nature in love, and this plot does
not present sentimentality but only the connection
between love and transcendence.

The desired body articulates desire in promise, a passage
from the language of vision to that of touch, of
exhilaration, of the ecstasy of participation.

Even in failure, we know love; in the experience of love,
we are all Adam and Eve on the first day of creation
because the experience of others does not teach us love.

It does not teach us that love is the way of life or that this
way is beyond possibilities of human nature.

Who can open the way to transcendence if not love?

Love, the jealous guardian of the ultimate questions,
perhaps also guards the solution to this puzzle.

It is an enigma in which God sees the love for his nature,
the intertwining which creates does not host sentimentality
but only the connection between love and transcendence
that the mystics;

They have been able to capture the raptures of the soul.

When we define God as love, the drama of the Christian theology of the Four opens:

God, man, angel, and devil are linked in that cosmic event in which love is reflected.

In liberty and freedom, man finds his limit.

Man can never identify with the devil, with the guardian of the limit, and therefore he looks to death as to the dissolution of every limit, which is why we have always felt a kinship between love and death.

In concluding this exploration into the art of love, inspired by myths, authors, and artists, we find that love is a dynamic, ever-evolving masterpiece. From understanding desire's unconscious roots to embracing vulnerability, the chapters have illuminated the multifaceted nature of human connection.

This journey urged readers to view love as a skill—an art form requiring practice, patience, and continual growth. Each chapter, from unraveling desire to balancing power dynamics, contributed to the intricate canvas of understanding and mastering the art of love.

As we navigate this tapestry of emotions, it becomes clear that love is not a static destination but an ongoing expedition. The Eternal Flame reminds us to adapt, learn, and nurture our connections. Crafting a Love Manifesto empowers individuals to articulate their unique vision, fostering intentional relationships.

In the end, this book encourages readers to embrace love not merely as an emotion but as an art—one that, like any masterpiece, demands dedication, creativity, and the willingness to evolve. May this exploration guide you in sculpting a love that withstands the test of time—a living testament to the perpetual beauty of the ever-evolving art of love.

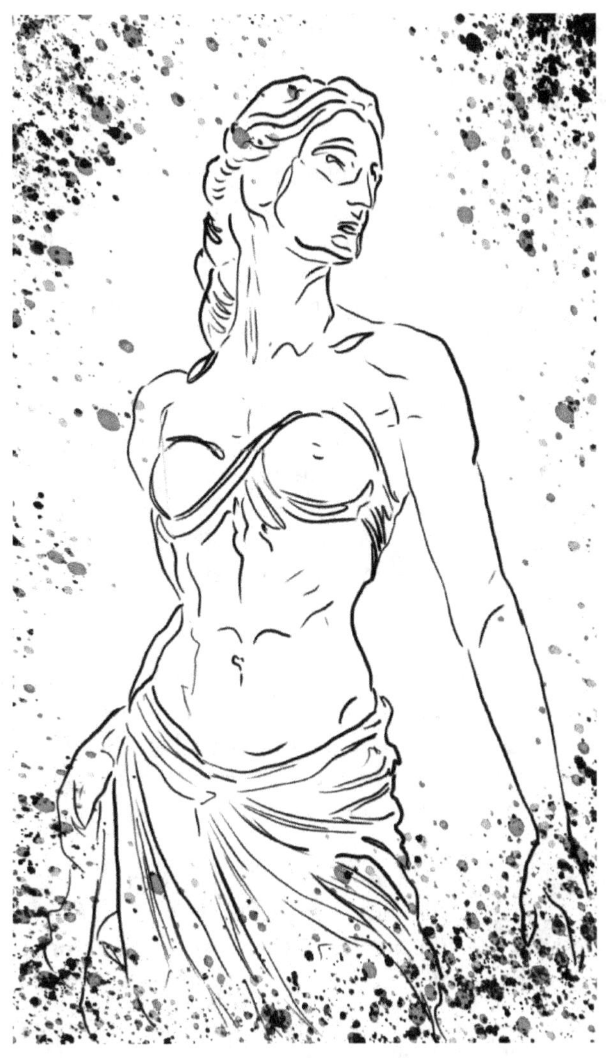

Shadow

The integration of shadows can empower individuals to engage in conscious and disciplined behavior to finally embrace their own path and role into society.

Epilogue: becoming a Love Master

Dear Reader;

As you close the final chapter of this exploration into the art of love, it's with great joy and fulfillment that we declare you a "love master." You've embarked on a journey inspired by the insights of Freud and Fromm, and through each chapter, you've delved into the complexities, nuances, and beauty of human connection.

By decoding desires, embracing vulnerability, and mastering the arts of touch and balance, you've acquired the wisdom needed to navigate the art of love. Your commitment to continuous growth, coupled with the crafting of your personal love manifesto, signifies a profound understanding of the ever-evolving nature of love.

As a love master, you've not only absorbed the lessons but internalized them, making them an intrinsic part of your approach to relationships. Your journey has transformed you into an artist, sculpting connections with intention, patience, and genuine care.

Remember, the art of love is a perpetual masterpiece, and as a love master, you hold the brush to shape enduring, meaningful relationships. May your love story continue to unfold as a testament to the mastery you've achieved.

With heartfelt congratulations,

Ricardo Sanchez, author and love master

ABOUT THE AUTHOR

Ricardo Sanchez, an Italian-Spanish artist who has become a citizen of the United States, commits himself to exploring and pondering the essence of love. He passionately embraces his role as a conduit for divine illumination, fervently striving to impart his insights to audiences through various forms of artistic expression, ranging from literature to show entertainment with his parallel musician-performer career.

www.ingramcontent.com/pod-product-compliance
Lightning Source LLC
Chambersburg PA
CBHW070904250726
48662CB00003B/1496